W9-BYZ-899

"One of the best books on the subject . . . emphasizes the positive aspects of menopause as a liberating transition to the next phase of life and offers sensible, empowering advice for women. Highly recommended."
—*Library Journal*

In *The Pause,* Lonnie Barbach revolutionizes menopause—just as she revolutionized female sexuality with her groundbreaking work on sex and intimacy in *For Yourself* and *For Each Other*. Drawing on first hand testimony from hundreds of women and the most up-to-the-minute medical research available, Lonnie Barbach provides invaluable guidance to help us feel in control, to empower us to make informed choices about the options facing us, and to let us fully understand and experience this major turning point, not with fear and discomfort but with strength, confidence, and glowing good health. You'll discover:

♦ Herbal remedies and vitamin supplements that work for PMS and menopause-related difficulties

♦ Ways to benefit from hormones while you're still menstruating

♦ Dozens of remedies for hot flashes and headaches

♦ Explicit suggestions to ease sexual difficulties—and make sex even better than ever

♦ How to handle physicians who may not offer the information or help you need

THE PAUSE

Lonnie Barbach, Ph.D.

the
pause

Positive Approaches
to Menopause

NEWLY REVISED AND UPDATED

Foreword by John Arpels, M.D.

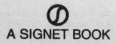

A SIGNET BOOK

PUBLISHER'S NOTE

The ideas, procedures and suggestions contained in this book are not intended as a substitute for consulting with your physician. All matters regarding your health require medical supervision.

Published by the Penguin Group
Penguin Books USA Inc., 375 Hudson Street,
New York, New York 10014, U.S.A.
Penguin Books Ltd, 27 Wrights Lane,
London W8 5TZ, England
Penguin Books, Australia Ltd, Ringwood,
Victoria, Australia
Penguin Books Canada Ltd, 10 Alcorn Avenue,
Toronto, Ontario, Canada M4V 3B2
Penguin Books (N.Z.) Ltd, 182-190 Wairau Road,
Auckland 10, New Zealand

Penguin Books Ltd, Registered Offices:
Harmondsworth, Middlesex, England

Published by Signet, an imprint of Dutton Signet, a division of Penguin Books USA Inc. Previously published in a Dutton edition.

First Signet Printing, April, 1994
10 9 8 7 6 5 4

Copyright © Lonnie Barbach, 1993
All rights reserved

*For my dear friend Jeri Marlowe,
who was the inspiration for this book.*

ACKNOWLEDGMENTS

This book could have never been written without the contributions of numerous health professionals. To begin with, John Arpels, M.D., gynecologist and specialist in menopause, gave me hours and hours of his time, patiently explaining concepts ranging from the simple to the most complex. His unique understanding of the field is reflected in the sections dealing with traditional medical interventions.

I would also especially like to thank Harriet Beinfield, L.Ac., acupuncturist, San Francisco; Bruce Ettinger, M.D., osteoporosis specialist, Kaiser Permanente, San Francisco; JoAnn Hattner, R.D., clinical dietitian, Stanford Medical School; Anna Harvey, D.C., chiropractor and herbalist, Mill Valley, California; Ifeoma Ikenze, M.D., homeopath, Kentfield, California; Patricia T. Kelly, Ph.D., medical geneticist, Los Angeles; Efrem Korngold, L.Ac., O.M.D., acupuncturist, San Francisco; Victoria Maclin, M.D., reproductive endocrinologist, Rush Medical College, Chicago; Norma

McCoy, Ph.D., psychologist, San Francisco State University; Scott Nelson, Ph.D., psychologist, Mill Valley, California; Martin L. Rossman, M.D., acupuncturist, Mill Valley, California; Richard Schmidt, M.D., urologist, University of California, San Francisco; Barbara Sherwin, Ph.D., psychologist, McGill University, Montreal, Quebec; Meir Stampfer, M.D., Ph.D., epidemiologist, Harvard Medical School, Boston; and Dana Ullman, M.P.H., homeopath, Berkeley, California. Each of these health professionals was kind enough to answer my questions whenever I called and to check the relevant sections of the manuscript for accuracy.

In addition, Gloria Bachmann, M.D.; Patricia Baldwin, R.N., N.P.; Stanley Birge, M.D.; Sharon de Buren, N.P.; Graham Colditz, M.D.P.H.; Winnifred B. Cutler, Ph.D.; Barbara Drinkwater, Ph.D.; Frederika Ebel-Riehl; Ricardo Fernandez, M.D.; Julie Freiberg, N.P., L.Ac.; Jan Gibbs, R.N.; Mark Glasser, M.D.; Sadja Greenwood, M.D.; Sonia Hamburger, B.A.; Joel Hargrove, M.D.; Jordan Horowitz, M.D.; Jifan Hu, Ph.D.; Greggory Johnson, P.T.; Helen Singer Kaplan, M.D., Ph.D.; Michael Klaper, M.D.; Albert Kligman, M.D.; Fredi Kronenberg, Ph.D.; Sandra Leiblum, Ph.D.; Edward M. Lichten, M.D.; Roger Lobo, M.D.; Chris Longcope, M.D.; Ed Lufkin, M.D.; Robert Marcus, M.D.; William Masters, M.D.; Bruce McEwen, M.D.; Kathryn Morris, M.D.; Mary Moss, R.N., N.P.; Lila Nachtigall, M.D.; Frederick Naftolin, M.D.; Morris Notelowitz, M.D., Ph.D.; Robert Phelps, M.D.; Malcom Powell, M.D.; Quentin Regestein, M.D.; Jacqueline Sa; Susan Schiffman, Ph.D.; David Shefrin, N.D.; Leon Speroff, M.D.; Sandra Swain, M.D.; Maida Taylor, M.D.; Wolf Utian, M.D.; Joyce Venis, R.N.C.; Roland Young, M.D.; and Ed Zelniker, Ph.G., all gave generously of their time and knowledge. I could not have done the book without them.

The life of the book really came from all of the women

who took the time to share with me the joys and hardships of their personal transitions through menopause. Many even continued to telephone periodically to keep me apprised of the results of their most recent experiences.

My dear friend, Donna Rosenthal, who edited the book for me, was masterful in her observations and criticism. Marilyn Anderson, who typed each revision of the manuscript and organized all of the reference material, remained enthusiastic throughout. She generously gave up her weekends and probably her eyesight to see this project completed. I would also like to thank Carolyn Rice for typing up all of my interviews with incredible speed and accuracy, and Don Ciccone for his unending searches of the medical literature.

I so much appreciate Carole DeSanti, my editor at Dutton, and Rhoda Weyr, my agent, both of whom provided essential feedback and encouragement.

I could never have completed this book with any semblance of sanity without the support of David L. Geisinger, the love of my life. His patience was unending, his meals delicious, and his chapter titles inspired. And, of course, I cannot forget to mention our daughter, Tess, who managed to brighten even those days when work was most grueling.

CONTENTS

FOREWORD

In the next ten years more women will be going through menopause, entering their hormone transition years, than in all of recorded history. Women over fifty will account for fully 25 percent of the world's population in slightly more than thirty years.

This book has been written especially for you. In a sense it has also been written *by* you. The voices of all Lonnie Barbach's friends and patients heard herein are a unified chorus of needs, fears, and hopes—a clear expression of the experiences women share at this watershed in their lives. The transition through menopause exists. The symptoms are real, the discomfort not imagined, the trepidations valid. Though this voyage is one not taken by 49 percent of the population—we the men, who dominate the pinnacles of business and the ivory towers of medicine— women deserve to be heard, and to be equipped for the journey with the facts. It doesn't come any more factual than here in *The Pause*.

This wonderful book contains all the questions asked and all the symptoms felt. All the answers may not be found here only because until recently women have not been taken seriously enough to generate the necessary studies. We still have much to learn, but much is already known. This book presents what is known, in a simple and concise format applicable to all women.

The discussion of PMS and how female hormones interact with various brain functions is state of the art information. It encompasses very sophisticated research data which shows that the biological network of brain circuits controlling emotion, memory, sex drive, and temperature regulation needs estrogen to stay wired together properly. Lonnie Barbach has taken information gleaned from psychological profile studies which show that women low in estrogen greatly improve their scores for both mood and memory when given adequate estrogen replacement, and applied this to the available neuroendocrinology findings. The final outcome is the most advanced clinically relevant discussion anywhere to be found on why women feel good when their hormones are in sync and why they feel rotten when things go awry.

The Pause contains information on the cutting edge of menopausal medicine, which, it's hoped, will lead to useful remedies for all women who need or want such information. This book explores not only what happens during the transitional years but also *why* these bothersome events occur. *The Pause* offers you the best sort of knowledge: the certainty that you are normal and the comprehension of what is going on inside you.

Equally unique is Lonnie's gentle blend of treatments taken from both traditional medicine and holistic disciplines such as homeopathy, acupuncture, and herbal pharmacopoeia.

Finally, *The Pause* offers wise words for men. For at times the best medicine of all can be a simple "I understand," from a comforting partner, family member, or friend.

As you will learn from the testimony of the women quoted here, menopause can herald a time of renewal and fresh achievement. At this vital transition in your life, the insights of *The Pause* should prove invaluable.

—John C. Arpels, M.D., founding member,
North American Menopause Society;
Associate Clinical Professor,
Department of Obstetrics and Gynecology,
University of California at San Francisco

What Is "The Pause"?

1

Knowledge Is Power

It was September 1987, a month before my forty-third birthday. My life was going well. My daughter was nearly two years old and except for her erratic sleeping patterns was a total delight. David was a supportive, wonderful partner. I was excited about finishing my first videotape, *Falling in Love Again*, when suddenly the rug was pulled out from under me.

I began feeling so fatigued that I was forced to take a nap each afternoon. Certainly being the working mother of a two-year-old can be exhausting, but this fatigue was different. I felt the way I had during the first three months of my pregnancy, but then I knew the cause. In addition to the fatigue, I was having strange heart palpitations, and I was waking up three to five times a night to urinate. One of my fingernails constantly felt cold and a vertebra in my neck was suspiciously tender.

By the morning of the final shoot for the videotape, instead of feeling like celebrating, I wanted to crawl into a hole. I did not know whether I would be able to make it through the day. All I knew was that there was something terribly wrong with me.

In the following year I trekked from doctor to doctor, trying to find the cause of these strange symptoms. One physician thought I had chronic fatigue syndrome and another suggested systemic candida. Since I could not do anything about chronic fatigue syndrome, I chose systemic candida as my diagnosis and religiously followed a strict diet, free of yeast, wheat, and sugar. In four months, I lost fifteen pounds, looked awful, and still felt terrible.

Yet another doctor diagnosed me as having low thyroid. My blood tests showed that I was on the very low end of normal. I was given thyroid medication, the minimum dose. Even when I cut the dose in half and then in half again, I could not sleep more than three hours a night and I shook as if I had been mainlining coffee. So my thyroid was not the problem.

During that year, my menstrual cycles had shortened to twenty-eight days from the usual thirty-one to thirty-three. I even had a couple of twenty-six-day cycles and one that was just twenty-one days long. But I thought this irregularity was the *result* of my mysterious illness rather than the cause of it. All I could think of was Gilda Radner, dying of ovarian cancer, which none in her parade of doctors had diagnosed until it was too late.

I remained confused and frustrated for more than a year. Then one morning I took a walk with a friend, two years my senior. She informed me that the strange symptoms *she* had been experiencing were menopause and that maybe that was my problem.

Menopause? Me? No way! That couldn't be what I was going through—I was too young. I had no idea that symptoms could begin before age fifty. In fact, except for hot

flashes, I did not know there were any symptoms at all—
and I had never had a hot flash.

My immediate fear was that my years of productivity
were over. Not reproductivity, but productivity. I love my
work as psychologist, author, and lecturer. I couldn't imagine it all ending. During the next few weeks, I began to do
some serious thinking. I had at least two decades before retirement age, which meant I had as many productive years
ahead as I had behind. In fact, my increased life experience was making my work deeper and better. As I reflected, I realized that menopause did not have to mean
the beginning of the end of my life. Instead, it could mark
the beginning of a powerful and productive time. I was actually at the height of my career.

I discovered that my fears and ignorance were not
unique. A successful TV producer told me that at forty-six,
she was puzzled by strange symptoms. Her periods were so
heavy she had to use a "super" Tampax plus two pads.
The periods were accompanied by excessive cramping and
fatigue and she often felt crabby and on the edge of anger.
But when I suggested that her symptoms could be signs of
the beginning of her menopausal transition, she was devastated, just as I had been. "Oh no, I'm not ready for this,"
she said. "I have so much left to accomplish and I'm having a wonderful life." When I asked her what part of her
life had been the best, she replied, "The last few years,
without a doubt, both in my marriage and my career."
With menopause, she expected it all to end.

My personal experiences led me to write *The Pause*. I
wanted to create a more realistic picture of menopause
and help dispel the notion that it means we are somehow
finished or washed up when it occurs. I also wanted to
provide information on the variety of early signs and
symptoms of menopause so that others will not have to go
through the emotional distress that lack of information

caused me. And finally, I wanted to direct women experiencing uncomfortable symptoms toward traditional and alternative approaches to ameliorating them. Basically, I found myself writing the book that I wished had prepared me for this passage.

With guidance and preparation, this transition can be as exciting as pregnancy. This episode in our lives can truly be thought of as a period of gestation, culminating in our own rebirth. This is a time of *renewal,* not the beginning of death. For this reason, I would like to start by renaming this phase of women's lives. We need to overcome the many negative expectations that surround the word "menopause." What shall we call it?

"The change of life" is imposing and can easily be misinterpreted as the change from life to death. "The perimenopause," which is the proper medical term for the years of hormonal change preceding menopause, is just too unwieldy. I cannot imagine talking to a friend about my "perimenopausal" experience. While I like the meaning of the term "climacteric" (a major turning point or critical stage), it is awkward and somehow sounds like a climax that has not yet happened.

"The Pause" really fits the most positive aspects of the experience for me. It speaks of a break, a time to reflect. This transition from our childbearing years to the next stage of life, in which our own needs can play a more central part in the story that unfolds, promises excitement.

It's sort of like pushing the pause button on your VCR player: you take a break for a few minutes to answer the phone or scoop out some frozen yogurt. You can do a lot of things during this interlude, but ultimately you expect to continue from where you left off. Or maybe the pause offered by a sabbatical is a better analogy. You take time out from the routine of your life. You encounter new experiences—often altering your point of view. Then you return to life as usual—the same person, yet somehow changed because of it all. While The Pause may be a period of disequilibrium, of physical discomfort, it also heralds a new equilibrium, a period of renewed energy, and often a new sense of purpose.

I use "The Pause" to refer to the period of discomfort that precedes the last menstrual cycle and often continues for a few months to a couple of years thereafter. "Menopause," on the other hand, refers *specifically* to the date of the last menstrual period, and "postmenopause" addresses the years after that date.

Many physicians simply do not understand that the transition to menopause is a process that can take years. The Pause can start as soon as our late thirties or early forties. The number of women who reported that their gynecologists told them that their symptoms had nothing to do with menopause because they were not yet fifty was simply astounding.

"With my yearly physical, I'd ask for information about menopause and I'd get a pat on the back and an, 'Oh, don't worry about that until you're fifty-two.' "

"When I was forty-five, I was having horrible headaches, my periods were growing further apart and I was flowing heavily. I asked if there wasn't a test I could take to find out if it was menopause. But the doctor said that it was all in my head, that I was too young, it couldn't be."

"In my early forties I was having these terrible mood swings so I made an appointment with my gynecologist, but he said I was too young for menopause and I shouldn't think any more about it."

In the two to ten years *before* the last menstrual period, and the year or so after, women tend to experience the most difficult physical and emotional symptoms. If you are between thirty-eight and forty-five and going through this transition, doctors may ignore you—you may feel awful, but can't find out why.

> "I was forty-two years old. I was starting to get these un-
> usual headaches, a kind of numbness in one of my fingers,
> and incredible fatigue. I didn't know what it was and no
> doctor seemed to be able to provide me with a diagnosis.
> What really scared me at the time was that these were the
> cardinal symptoms of a brain tumor. It turned out to be
> menopause."

It is not knowing, maybe more than anything, that holds women in the grip of fear. Had I known at the time that the physical problems I was experiencing were classic signs of menopause, I could have saved the time, money, and grief of visiting doctors. Not knowing the cause of my symptoms made it more difficult for me to deal with the physiological discomfort. For this reason, I have devoted Chapters 3 through 6, one chapter each, to the different constellations of emotional and physical symptoms that may accompany The Pause. Besides describing the various symptoms, I cover traditional and alternative solutions when appropriate. Chapter 7 deals specifically with the sexual changes that can occur during this period of our lives.

With the dearth of information available to women, and the covert whisperings about what it all means, we find ourselves anxious and ignorant about a normal process that takes place within *every* woman who lives beyond her middle fifties. Chapter 2 describes this process simply and clearly. A postmenopausal woman is no more hormonally deficient than a girl of six with no breasts. Each is normal for a female of that age. Like puberty and childbirth—

each with its own pleasures and problems—menopause is a normal and natural transition.

It is more appropriate to look at The Pause and the postmenopausal period in the same way we view handling the reproductive period. We do not consider pregnancy a disease, although we may call upon medical support and guidance to help us through. If we have problems, intervention is appropriate. If not, nature takes its course.

In the same way, not every woman needs to be treated when going through The Pause. Many will experience virtually no distress whatsoever or only mild symptoms. However, when we experience symptoms related to The Pause, many of us do not know where to turn. One major concern is whether or not to take hormones.

The decision to take or not to take hormones reflects our individual approach to health care. Consequently, the pros and cons of this very personal decision are covered in Chapter 8. That chapter also presents the most up-to-date medical information from the North American Menopause Society's annual meetings, and research findings from professional journals. Despite the large numbers of women going through menopause, it has not been given real medical attention until very recently. Only over the past four years has the North American Menopause Society been holding annual meetings to communicate new scientific information. Consequently, on a couple of issues there is still disagreement even among the experts, and there is still much that is not known.

In addition to standard hormone replacement therapy, I will explore the positive and negative aspects of low-dose birth control pills and estrogen supplementation in the forms of pills, the estrogen patch, or estrogen cream—solutions appropriate to women in their forties who are still menstruating. New forms of progesterone will also be covered. Your physician, especially if he or she does not specialize in menopause, may not yet be aware of some of these alternatives.

Hormones are not the only viable way to counter the discomforts of The Pause. Some women are wary of hormones or downright opposed to taking them. Others may have risk factors that do not permit them to take hormones. And many women prefer the least possible intervention or the most natural approach. For example, their first choice might be to do nothing at all, or to take vitamin supplements. Even when research is scanty or nonexistent, some women intuitively trust alternative therapies—herbs, homeopathy, or acupuncture—more than Western medicine.

Chapter 9 explores a number of alternative treatment approaches. Herbs that balance your hormones or contain phytosterols (natural plant hormones) can provide relief from symptoms. Homeopaths are physicians or other health professionals specifically trained to use specially prepared microdoses of herbs or other plants, minerals, or animal fluids to reduce discomfort. Acupuncturists rely on the use of needles or electrical stimulation of particular points in the body, often accompanied by Chinese herbs, to reequilibrate the energy flow in the body and alleviate symptoms. Each of these alternatives requires treatment by a specialist. This chapter discusses the benefits and limitations of each.

I do not favor one treatment modality over another. Each has different strengths, and I have tried most of them with some degree of success. The final decision lies in your particular risk factors, and the way your body responds to hormones, homeopathic remedies, acupuncture treatments, or herbs. It also depends on how you feel about the different methods, about taking daily pills, for example, as opposed to having acupuncture needles inserted into your body.

There is no one, right, risk-free answer. Every time you put something in your body you take a risk. You also take a risk when you do nothing, perhaps depriving your body of what it needs. And, no single approach works all the time for any particular symptom. Some women respond to some approaches, others to different ones. But relief *is* possible. When you have choices, you can chart your own course.

> "I'm really not afraid of getting old or losing my childbearing years. Still, I had problems with menopause. If I had known that I could change things with vitamins or homeopathy or something, I would have been better off. When you have no knowledge, you have no alternative."

Most of us would like to make our transit through The Pause as painless as possible, but many of us are as much concerned about our health in the years that lie beyond. Chapter 10 is devoted to the prevention of heart disease and osteoporosis, to living the most healthful lives we can. The roles of hormones, diet, and exercise are all explored. Diet and exercise are also addressed in other sections where relevant.

My goal in *The Pause* is to provide you with appropriate alternatives for handling your symptoms, whether they are hardly noticeable or overwhelming, including alternatives for minimizing future health problems. With information comes power, power to seek the care you need. Without information, you do not know the appropriate questions to ask and are at the mercy of your health practitioner. Information is the tool for judging whether you are receiving the best care possible.

For most of you, The Pause is unlikely to be as difficult as you may anticipate. Much like a steep ski slope, it generally looks far worse from above. Once in the middle, you can find a way down. Research shows that women who experienced regret or mixed feelings at the beginning of The Pause were likely to change their minds in a positive direction. And those who felt relieved at the start of The Pause *continued* to feel that way.

Even when the transition is difficult, the rewards can be great. Some of the most beautiful landscapes are accessible only after a rugged climb.

As one woman said to me: "If I did a new résumé, I think I'd put down, 'I went through menopause,' because it means something. I see it as another form of accomplishment. I went through it my own way, and I came out the other side. And I am a better person for it. "

Menopause is not the end of your life; it is the beginning of a new phase. Knowledge of what is to come can empower you to make this phase into the best one of all, and Chapter 11 shows you how women have done just this.

2

The Process
of
"The Pause"

So you've been feeling a bit tired lately. Maybe it's because you've been waking up a few times at night and having difficulty getting back to sleep. Or it's possible you don't feel quite well—nothing you can put your finger on, just feeling a bit down or irritable; maybe things just seem to upset you more easily these days. And come to think of it, your periods have changed a bit. Nothing remarkable; in fact, it's hardly noticeable. But your cycle *is* a bit longer or shorter and the bleeding somewhat lighter or heavier than usual.

But you're only in your early to mid-forties, maybe just your late thirties. It *couldn't* be the beginning of The Pause, could it? Yes, it could.

While in rare cases a woman's periods just suddenly end one day, most women find that the process of The Pause averages between two and ten years, and can sometimes take as long as fifteen. One woman I interviewed started having irregular cycles when she was thirty-six. She was having a period every two or three weeks and they were lasting ten to fourteen days. It seemed as if she was bleeding all the time. When she had her hormone levels tested, they were all over the map. She had a series of D&Cs—a scraping of the uterus frequently done when there is irregular bleeding with no known cause. Her gynecologist hoped that removing the top layer of cells from the uterine lining would address the cause of the bleeding and it would stop. When one doctor *did* label her symptoms menopause, she left his office in a huff. She could not believe he would even intimate such a thing. Finally, when she was forty-eight, her periods stopped completely. For her, menopause was a difficult and drawn-out process.

Just as each woman experiences pregnancy differently, we each go through The Pause in our own fashion. Some women breeze through pregnancy and then further infuriate the rest of us with a three-hour labor and delivery. Others have no problems in the early stages of pregnancy, but end up spending the last three months in bed or require a C-section. And some women remain sick from the moment they conceive and are further tormented by postpartum depression. With menopause, women range from having virtually no symptoms except the cessation of their periods to suffering symptoms that severely interfere with day-to-day living.

Many of our reactions, both to pregnancy and to The Pause, have to do with the intensity of hormonal changes and our sensitivity to them. To begin with, we each have unique levels of hormones coursing through our bodies, causing menstrual cycles ranging from twenty-six to thirty-two days. In addition, our different diets, exercise patterns, and life experiences make us more and more unlike one another as we age. Add to this the different ways in which the hormonal changes take place during this period, from abrupt drops and surges to a gradual tapering off of hor-

mone production, and you can see how the process of The
Pause can be infinitely variable.

Furthermore, some of us are more sensitive to our fluctuating hormones than others. The same absolute hormonal change that creates symptoms in one woman will
hardly be noticed by another. And a level of symptoms experienced by one woman may cause her to seek medical
intervention, while another with the same physical symptoms might grin and bear it.

Finally, the ease or difficulty with which we are visited
by The Pause is further affected by factors such as stress,
diet, smoking, genetic differences, and individual or cultural attitudes toward menopause. Japanese women, for
example, don't have hot flashes; they have stiff shoulders.
Mayan women express virtually no physical complaints at
all. In contrast, women in a number of African tribes report complaints very similar to those of Western women.

Unfortunately, women who are the most likely candidates for problems with menopause are those who have
experienced premenstrual syndrome (PMS) or postpartum
depression. These are the women who tend to be most
sensitive to hormonal fluctuations.

"At sixteen I'd come home from school because I'd be terribly depressed and I'd have such bad cramps I'd feel sick.
And I remember they always told me: 'As you get older, it
gets better.' Then they said, 'When you have kids, it all goes
away.' Well, I got older and I had kids and it never went
away. And now I'm going through menopause and I'm still
complaining about it."

It appears that 10 to 15 percent of women breeze
through The Pause with virtually no discomfort.

"I'm fifty-two and to me, menopause really never was a big
issue. I don't have my periods anymore. That stopped when

I was forty-nine. First the timing of my periods was weird, they didn't come on time, but I never bled like some women. I never really had any problems. I occasionally have hot flashes, but by no means do I pay much attention to it."

"I'll be forty-eight next week. I'm just beginning menopause because every once in a while I miss a period. I also find that I have to exercise more to keep from gaining weight and I don't think it's because I've changed the way I've been eating, but that's about all I've noticed."

Another 10 to 15 percent of women experience symptoms so severe they are incapacitated.

"Though I am normally even-tempered, I started to have psychotic experiences. I felt enraged, out of control. I was having hot flashes that felt like panic attacks every twenty minutes—day and night. I couldn't work. Most of the time, I couldn't even be around people."

"I've been a person who always felt well. But over the last five or six years, it's been yuck. I've even thought, 'What's the purpose of living?' because the quality of my life has been so bad—fighting constantly at work, with myself, with my body."

Women who experience a difficult menopause are often dismissed as neurotic or hypochondriacal. Unfortunately, many of us accept this label, especially if we do not know others who are suffering similarly.

"I used to think that women who had problems with menopause had the problem up in their heads. I knew it would be a breeze for me. Boy, was I ever surprised when I had these vicious hot flashes and unbelievable mood swings. It really taught me humility."

What are symptoms women commonly experience during The Pause? They include night awakenings, headaches, joint pains, unusual skin sensitivities, fatigue, irritability, moodiness, memory loss, mental sluggishness, hot flashes, and night sweats. Some women also feel a lack of sexual desire, lack of vaginal lubrication, and pain with intercourse. The good news is you are unlikely to get *all* of these symptoms. The bad news is none of them is fun. But remember, symptoms for most of us are mild, not sufficient to disrupt the daily routine seriously, especially once we realize that they are a response to The Pause and nothing more.

"It's so subtle, it really sneaks up on you. I had a hard time sleeping at night. I would get hot flashes and wake up drenched. And my sexual interest did go down a bit."

Maybe the best way to explain why we experience symptoms is first to describe the process our bodies undergo during our reproductive years, and then to show how it changes as we enter The Pause.

"It's like making popcorn," says Dr. Jordan Horowitz, a San Francisco obstetrician and gynecologist. "Imagine the eggs as corn kernels and the hormones as heat. During puberty the eggs are all there. But it's not until the hormones are turned up that periods begin. Most young women are prone to irregular ovulation for a while, much like the first kernels of popcorn that go off intermittently. In the middle of reproductive life, like the middle of the popcorn analogy, we see regular ovulation and regular popping. But as you have fewer kernels left, they again pop more irregularly. In fact, just before all the kernels have popped, there may be a quiet moment when you think everything's finished. Then suddenly a few more kernels pop. That is what happens as you get close to menopause. You may have a few months without ovulation and suddenly you'll ovulate again, until finally, everything that is going to pop has popped. And then you have reached menopause."

THE HORMONIC SYMPHONY

Now let's see how hormones figure into this popcorn analogy. Basically, your hormones regulate one another in a complex feedback system resembling a thermostat. When the temperature in your house reaches a certain low level, the thermostat signals the heater to turn on. Once the temperature is high enough, the thermostat turns the heater off. Your hormones signal each other in a similar way. There are actually a number of different hormones involved in the menstrual cycle, but for the sake of simplicity, we'll stick with the major players: estrogen, progesterone, FSH (follicle-stimulating hormone), and LH (luteinizing hormone).

Let's imagine a hypothetical twenty-eight-day cycle. On day 1, you start bleeding. At this point, estrogen and progesterone are at their lowest level. (Take my word for it; you'll see why later.) Once these hormones reach this low level, the thermostat turns on and signals the pituitary to begin producing FSH, follicle-stimulating hormone. FSH encourages the follicles in the ovary to ripen. A follicle is an egg surrounded by a layer of hormone-producing cells.

Initially, FSH causes a number of follicles to develop, but generally only one, the dominant follicle, called the Graafian follicle, will mature to ovulation. (One way we get twins or triplets is when more than one egg matures.) As the follicles are developing, they each secrete estrogen. Among other things, the estrogen causes blood to be brought to the uterine lining to prepare it for the implantation of the egg.

For the first twelve days of the cycle, FSH and estrogen levels are rising. Once the estrogen level is high enough, the thermostat signals the pituitary to stop producing FSH, and to start secreting more LH, luteinizing hormone. This midcycle surge of LH causes the egg to be released from the Graafian follicle. This is called ovulation and occurs at about day 14.

The empty follicle is now called the corpus luteum, or yellow body. This yellow body secretes its own estrogen and progesterone. Progesterone is the hormone that matures the uterine lining created by the estrogen and prepares it for pregnancy. Another thermostat begins working, and when the progesterone reaches a sufficiently high level, it signals the pituitary to shut off production of LH.

Even though FSH and LH have been shut off, the corpus luteum keeps pumping out estrogen and progesterone until about day 22, when it runs out of steam. If fertilization occurs, the fertilized egg begins secreting hormones of its own. If not, levels of progesterone and estrogen just keep decreasing. This rapid decline of estrogen and progesterone, which occurs about five to seven days before menstruation begins, produces premenstrual symptoms in many women.

Deprived of estrogen and progesterone, the blood vessels in the uterine wall (which has been prepared for the implantation of the fertilized egg) go into spasm and contract. This causes the uterine lining to break down and the blood cells and mucus that make up the lining are shed, and bleeding begins.

Now you are back to day 1, when the low levels of estrogen and progesterone trip the thermostat and signal the pituitary to begin releasing FSH—and the cycle begins again.

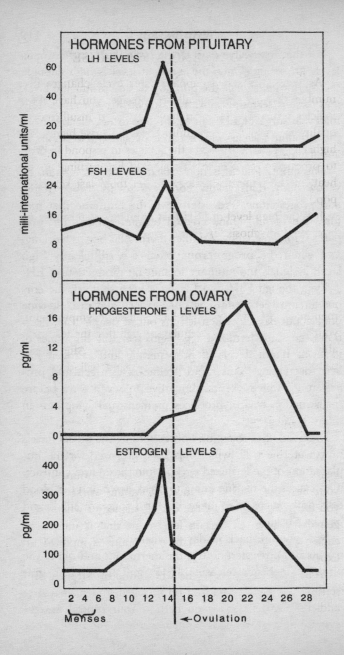

APPROACHING MENOPAUSE

As you approach menopause this cycle changes in a number of ways. First of all, as you age, you have fewer follicles left and those you have are often insufficient in quality to make it to ovulation. FSH levels rise higher and higher in an attempt to get the follicles to respond in order to produce a good egg. (It's kind of like turning up the heat, in the popcorn analogy, to get those last kernels to pop.)

It is the high level of FSH that ultimately determines the hormonal diagnosis of menopause. Unfortunately, FSH testing is often not diagnostically helpful because many women experience uncomfortable symptoms long before their FSH level rises to any degree. And by the time your FSH level rises above 40, the official determination of menopause, you are likely to have sufficient symptoms and your periods should be irregular enough that the test probably only confirms what you already know. After menopause, this FSH level will stay high and will drop only slightly over the years.

Disequilibrium

What you have during The Pause, those two to ten years before your periods stop, is disequilibrium. When your hormones are in balance, everything works well and you feel fine. When they are out of balance or when estrogen drops below a certain level—one that is unique for each woman and detected by her brain—symptoms are experienced.

Your body responds to the withdrawal of estrogen. In a sense, your body is hooked on estrogen, much as a drug addict's body is hooked on heroin. Your central nervous system and other bodily functions have become accustomed to operating with certain levels of estrogen. When the estrogen drops below this comfort level, called the estrogen set-point, you experience symptoms just as the drug addict does when heroin is withheld. However, once you adapt to the lowered levels of estrogen (like after a drug addict has withdrawn from a drug), symptoms stop.

The problem is that you are not being withdrawn from estrogen in a steady and gradual manner. For example, in some months during The Pause you may have a "good" ovulation, and your estrogen level surges. This is like interrupting a drug addict's withdrawal program with a fix from time to time. The additional estrogen creates new receptors which produce symptoms when they are again deprived of estrogen as levels descend further.

COMMON PATTERNS

While we each go through The Pause in our own unique manner, there are a couple of fairly common patterns of hormone imbalance that can produce uncomfortable symptoms.

In the first pattern, estrogen levels are too high in relation to progesterone levels. This commonly occurs in midcycle as FSH and LH levels have been turned up in an attempt to stimulate one follicle to ovulate. Because the follicles are substandard, a number need to be stimulated, each one producing estrogen. This estrogen surge can lead to midcycle breast tenderness, headaches, nausea, and some bloating. You may also have heavy bleeding, or it may take a lot longer than the usual fourteen days to produce one good egg, thereby extending the cycle.

A second common pattern occurs during the second half of the menstrual cycle if progesterone levels are higher in comparison to estrogen levels. This happens when estrogen declines more rapidly than progesterone. The relatively higher levels of progesterone actually turn off estrogen receptors. This diminishes the usable estrogen, causing the estrogen levels effectively to dip below the set-point. When this occurs, we see such symptoms as PMS, mood swings, memory loss, food cravings (especially for sweets), and hot flashes.

As hormones continue to taper off, it is not uncommon for the proper balance between them to be regained for some time (although at reduced levels); you may find yourself in a honeymoon period, where symptoms decline for a few months or even a few years. For example, as the number of good follicles dwindles, fewer are left to produce estrogen, and this midcycle surge of estrogen quiets down. The relatively high levels of progesterone subside when you hit months in which you do not ovulate—called anovulatory cycles—because there is no corpus luteum to produce progesterone in the second half of the cycle.

It is this break in symptoms that often causes women to doubt that menopause is really upon them. One woman I interviewed experienced this hiatus and concluded: "It can't be my hormones, because I'm just fine now. It was probably just stress." A couple of months later she began wondering all over again.

Finally, as you progress further toward menopause, fewer and fewer follicles are capable of ovulation—the final stages of the popcorn analogy. As estrogen levels continue to decrease further, you may drop below the estrogen set-point for a greater portion of the month. Initially, it may just be the last week of the month; then it is the last half of the month. Finally, women who are sensitive to this estrogen set-point may be symptomatic most of the time.

However, after a period of time, with no more ovulations and no more intermittent surges of estrogen, you adapt to the lowered levels of hormones, and symptoms disappear permanently.

Premature and Surgical Menopause

The process I have described is that of a natural menopause. It generally begins for women during their forties, but it can start earlier. Most women *complete* menopause between ages forty-five and fifty-five. The age at which your mother went through menopause is a fairly good indicator of your probable age at menopause. However, certain factors can result in an earlier transition. Women who have never been pregnant and those who have had their uterus removed, as well as women who have been vegetarians or have been malnourished or anorexic for extended periods, are apt to go through menopause one to four years earlier than the average. But smoking, as it turns out, is the *major* cause of an early menopause. Tobacco not only induces premature aging in all areas, it has a toxic effect on the ovaries.

About 1 percent of women go through what is termed "premature ovarian failure," meaning that their periods stop completely *before* their fortieth birthday. Ovarian damage from radiation or chemotherapy, or from certain autoimmune disorders and genetic abnormalities, is the most common cause of premature ovarian failure.

Missing periods, even for an extended time, is not the same as premature menopause. Physical and emotional stress can and will affect our menstrual cycles. We know that anorexia nervosa—undereating to the point of extreme thinness—and unusual athletic training such as marathon running, or even changing time zones, can inhibit menstruation. Emotional stress such as a traumatic divorce or the death of a loved one can have the same effect. Generally, however, menstrual cycles will begin again once the stressful situation has ended.

Some women enter menopause as a result of an oophorectomy, the removal of the ovaries. This is called a surgical menopause. If just the uterus is removed, a woman still goes through a natural menopause at the appropriate time, but she may not recognize it right away because without a uterus she no longer has periods and so cannot use a change in her menstrual cycle as confirmatory evidence.

When the ovaries are removed, a woman goes through an abrupt menopause. Her FSH and LH rise dramatically within a very short time as all of the hormones produced by her ovaries are cut off overnight. As a result, she is likely to experience exaggerated symptoms—everything from intense hot flashes to a precipitous drop in sexual desire.

Despite a reduction in function, the ovaries continue to produce hormones long after menopause is completed. This is one of the reasons you do not want to have your ovaries removed unless absolutely necessary. Along with the adrenal glands, the ovaries produce androgens. One of the androgens, called testosterone, is primarily responsible for our sex drive.

Androstenedione, another androgen produced in both the ovaries and the adrenals, is converted into estrogen largely in our fat cells. Our fat cells act as miniature factories, changing androgens into estrogen. Women with a little extra fat have more estrogen. This is one reason why thinner women tend to experience more symptoms during The Pause. Over time, this process of converting androgens to estrogen in the fat cells gets more and more refined. So even after you have gone through menopause, you are not necessarily hormonally depleted. Many women continue to produce sufficient hormones to live perfectly comfortably on every level. Others experience sexual problems or are more likely candidates for heart disease or osteoporosis in later life.

A NEW BEGINNING

Once a natural menopause is reached, or at least within a couple of years *after* the last menstrual cycle, most women will have adapted to a lowered level of estrogen and, except in rare cases, most nonsexually related symptoms will have ceased. In fact, after menopause most women start to feel great. And they report fewer symptoms, both physical and psychological, than at any earlier time in their lives.

"One thing I've noticed is a difference in my energy level. It's incredible. There are no ups or downs like I used to have as I went through my cycle getting ready for my period. It's just leveled out. That's the thing I've noticed most; it's the best."

Menopause is like a tunnel. Some women flow through effortlessly. Others bounce back and forth off the walls. But eventually everyone gets through. The one thing to keep in mind during this time is that there is a light at the end of the tunnel. Menopause does conclude and positive changes await us at the other side.

Further Information

Sadja Greenwood, M.D. *Menopause Naturally.* Volcano, CA: Volcano Press, 1992.

Louis Jovanovic, M.D., and Genell J. Subak-Sharpe. *Hormones: The Woman's Answerbook.* New York: Fawcett Columbine, 1987.

II

Signs and
Solutions

3

Riding
the Emotional
Roller Coaster

How much of menopause is in our heads, our psychological reaction to the *meaning* of the physical changes we are experiencing? And how much of it is a direct effect of changing hormones on our brains and central nervous system?

There is no question that the idea of menopause has a major psychological impact. Having no more periods when you are not pregnant and not under stress or traveling is an unmistakable life change. And it makes us confront our own mortality in a real and undeniable way.

"When I realized I was going through menopause, I just assumed that I was going to die soon, or that I was going to become a wrinkled old prune."

"What is reflected is that you're going to be dried up, you're going to be undesirable, your life is over and you have nothing to look forward to. It's like the beginning of the end and you have to deal with all of those mortality issues, like am I living my life the way I want to."

It's interesting that unconsciously we continue to hold to the idea that menopause marks the end of our lives, while in reality, most of us are a far cry from death's door. If you are in your forties today, you can expect to live to about age eighty-one.

Still, in a culture in which youth is revered and age is feared, menopause becomes a stigma.

"When I was younger, I thought menopause was something to be ashamed of. If I heard a rumor that a woman was starting menopause, it was 'Hush, hush.' I'd say, 'How terrible.' I didn't even know what I was talking about, but I thought it was terrible."

Because of our own fears of aging and American society's negative view of menopause, we may deny our symptoms and look for some other explanations for the changes we are experiencing.

"I was really in denial about it, kind of a classic psychological denial. I didn't believe it. I thought my gynecologist was wrong. I thought you had to be at least in your fifties. I wasn't in menopause, I was under stress or something and my periods would come back. It was only after it was exceedingly obvious, when I had hot flashes and I hadn't had a period for over five months, that I finally accepted it for what it was."

Some of us feel that if we ignore The Pause, if we pretend it is not happening, it will go away. I met a friend at a party recently who was talking about her premenstrual mood swings, which were becoming more exaggerated. A few days earlier at work she had been so upset that she started crying and had to sneak down twelve flights of stairs so that no coworkers would see her swollen face as she left for home. When I talked to her about keeping a journal so that she could follow her symptoms precisely, she replied, "I don't think I can do that. I'd have to focus on it every day and it's something I don't even want to think about."

Research shows that premenopausal women have a much more negative view of menopause than women who have gone through it. Women who have experienced menopause discover there is nothing to fear. They have not turned into dried-up prunes; they have not lost their zest for life. Instead, most women find it just one more transition, neither harder nor easier than many others in life. After you have experienced menopause, the mystery lifts, and with knowledge come control and freedom from fear.

Different cultures seem to have different concerns regarding menopause. One study found that Muslim Arab women worried about decline in their partners' sexual interest because they were no longer fertile. Near Eastern Jews feared a decline in physical health, whereas European women were apprehensive about their mental health. As with European women, the major fear American women have about menopause is that they will lose control over their emotions and become hysterical and irrational.

PMS AND MENOPAUSE

Emotional upheavals are a common accompaniment to The Pause. A disequilibrium in hormones can produce a disequilibrium in emotions for many women. Premenstrual syndrome, or PMS, refers to a constellation of emotional and physical symptoms that affect approximately 60 percent of women to a mild or moderate degree and an additional 15–20 percent severely enough to disrupt optimal functioning at work and home. Emotionally, women suffering from PMS have mood swings and are depressed or irritable, easily angered or saddened. These symptoms are caused either by the relatively high progesterone levels or by the drop in estrogen that occurs during the last part of the cycle.

"It happened to me well before menopause ever started. About a week before my period I would get into a terrible mood. It would only last for a day or two, but when I realized it, I knew I'd get my period. I was really uptight, angry at everything for no good reason, and I'm not that kind of person."

"My husband can tell when my period is going to start, because of my mood. As I get about a week or closer to my period, I become a real bitch. I can't seem to control it."

As menopause approaches, many women who have never had PMS develop it. Others who have struggled with it for years may find their symptoms becoming more severe.

"I always feel frustrated before my period, but in the last year, it's started to get worse."

"I've gotten real morose leading up to my periods this last year. I've gotten to the point where I really feel just hopeless the day before. I never used to experience that."

"There are times I've been concerned that the depression wouldn't lift. It was lasting a week and I'd wake up in the morning crying. Then just as I was about to call a therapist, I would wake up and feel great. And then I would get my period."

"I've always had painful periods. In my case, when they called it the curse, they weren't kidding. And now it's menopause. I'm getting pretty fed up with these mood swings—yelling at my husband and being irrational with the kids."

It's one thing to have PMS symptoms that occur regularly. You can look at a calendar and prepare yourself. But as cycles become irregular, you often don't know what to pin your moods on, and you may feel more out of control.

"I've always had PMS very heavy for about two days before my period. It's been predictable for years. But now, having an irregular period means my feelings are less predictable and I don't know if it's my hormonal mood or what."

These mood swings can definitely be caused by reduced estrogen levels. According to Dr. John Arpels, "Whenever the level of estrogen drops below the set-point needed for the brain, emotional symptoms may occur. When a woman is twenty-eight, we call it PMS. When she is forty-five, we call it perimenopause. It's the same process. She just may experience these symptoms for a greater percentage of the month as the perimenopause progresses into menopause."

MOODINESS, IRRITABILITY, AND RAGE

Feeling moody for a few days before your period is one thing, but at least half of all American women, according to a number of studies, experience mood swings, anxiety, irritability, and even intermittent rage for most or all of the month as they get closer to menopause. It's common knowledge that teenagers, pregnant women, and women going through The Pause are unusually emotional. These are the three times in life when hormone fluctuations are at their greatest.

> "I have these unpredictable mood swings. I'll feel fine one minute, and all of a sudden I think my life is horrible and I can't see anything good about it."

> "I find myself crying at the drop of a hat."

"Impatience," "irritability," and "anger" were words frequently used by women I interviewed to describe their feelings.

> "I get crabby and angrier faster. God, I'm a bitch sometimes."

> "For the last three days, I've been waking up with a scowl on my face. It wasn't until today when I was back to normal that I realized that this is really frightening. I've felt as if I've had another person inside of me."

> "Even when I wasn't under stress, I would overreact. I'd find myself getting angry, shouting at my daughter, having a fight with my husband—and for no particular reason."

Sometimes this irritability results from the chronic sleep deprivation experienced by women as hot flashes or simply lowered estrogen levels cause them to awaken a number of times at night. For me, this irritability would feel like a kind of internal agitation, not too different from the feeling I sometimes have when I am extremely hungry. The problem was, eating wouldn't help. My good-natured, now five-year-old daughter would begin to mirror my bad mood. I started to have a glass of wine in the afternoon to soothe my nerves, and I began to understand how women can develop a dependence on alcohol during The Pause.

Irritability and lack of patience are particular problems for those of us who have teenagers who are traversing their own hormonal ups and downs. Collisions between mother and teenager are commonplace and often produce fireworks, yet mothering young children during this time, when patience runs thin, can also be particularly problematic. The strain of coping with a young child who is fascinated by a leaf when you are in a rush to get to the post office before it closes can be blown totally out of proportion when your hormones have already set your nerves on edge.

> "I'm in the unique category of being a woman in menopause who also has a five- and a two-year-old. Between the jitters, the sleeplessness and the mood swings, I've been a wreck. And it's not fair to them. I find myself screaming at the slightest provocation."

> "I have a three-and-a-half-year-old and my frustration threshold is very low. I'll yell at my son when he really didn't do anything terribly wrong. I feel out of control and then awful about myself, like I'm a total failure as a mother."

Feeling out of control is a big issue. Women just can't count on themselves to behave in their usual predictable ways. They get enraged, can't sleep, cry at Hallmark commercials.

> "The crying thing really bothers me a whole lot because I never know when a crying jag is going to come on."

> "You can count on yourself one day and then you can't the next. You never know what your state of mind is going to be like."

Some women feel uncharacteristically insecure for almost no reason. They have trouble making decisions or become overwhelmed with self-doubt.

"One day I was at a stop sign, at a small street, but I was afraid to drive across. I was paranoid, and this was simply not like me."

"I sometimes feel so anxious that I can't stay in a room with other people. I've stopped scheduling social engagements because I never know how I'm going to feel."

I am not normally insecure, but recently there have been days when I keep reliving certain interactions with friends, burdened with the fear that I have offended someone. However, when I've checked it out, I've found that no one noticed anything but me. It was all in my head. One day, when things were going just fine, I felt this insecurity well up. It was then that I knew for certain that my reactions were hormonally based. There was simply nothing in my life to pin it on. Sure enough, in a day or two the feelings were gone, and it was not because I had done anything to change them. They vanished as magically as they had appeared.

DEPRESSION

One study of 682 British women showed that depressed mood increased significantly during The Pause as compared to the premenopausal years. This depression may have a physical as well as a psychological basis.

The "empty nest" has been widely touted as a major cause of depression and psychological stress during The

Pause. Even women who have never had children may experience this time as one of significant mourning.

"Well, I've talked to a therapist as well as some of my friends about never being able to have a child. There's not a whole lot else you can do. Sometimes I feel depressed about it, and at other times I feel like I'm getting past it. I just try to come to terms with it, and think about other things I can do in my life."

"The one thing that bothers me the most about menopause is the fact that the choice to have children was taken from me. I may have chosen not to have children. Who knows. But because I went through menopause at thirty-nine, I was never given that choice."

"I would have liked to have had children, but menopause came very early. So I had to resign myself to the fact that I wouldn't."

Women who have had children may fantasize about having another one or two, but this is rarely more than a momentary consideration.

"Just as our son was about ready to go to college, my husband and I looked at each other and said, 'How come we didn't have more kids?' But that was the only time any ambivalence came up and it was brief."

"I went through a certain amount of mourning about the loss of a period of my life that had been very productive. I had to acknowledge to myself that I was losing that part of me. I said, 'Okay, grieve. There's nothing wrong with grieving. Then once you get through it, you can explore what's beyond.' "

Except for women who are infertile, or those who may have centered their entire lives around bearing and raising children, most women are only too happy to have their childbearing years over, to have their bodies back, to be freed from the encumbrances of birth control, and to have more time for themselves.

"Did it bother me not to be able to have children anymore? I couldn't have cared less. In fact, it was like, hooray."

Depression during The Pause can also be the result of feeling ill. Studies at the American Institute for Research in Cambridge, Massachusetts, show that women reporting at least two physical symptoms are about four times more likely to be depressed as women reporting no more than one symptom. The worse you feel physically and the more anxious you are about your physical health, the more likely you are to feel depressed. Some women also feel angry that the bodies they trust and depend on are letting them down. If there is no outlet for this anger, it can be turned inward and experienced as depression.

For many women, these feelings of depression are a direct result of lowered estrogen levels. It is a physiological rather than a psychological reaction to The Pause. One study that gives credence to diminished hormones as a cause for mild depression compared levels of depression among women who had had their uterus removed and those who had their ovaries removed as well. Both groups had undergone surgery and both had lost their ability to have children. However, the women who lost their ovaries—and, consequently, more of their hormones— evidenced significantly greater depression.

The way estrogen affects the brain and the central nervous system is far too complex to describe fully here. But estrogen levels do affect neurotransmitters, cerebral blood flow, and endorphins. Estrogen makes us feel good. Transsexuals undergoing sex-change operations who are

taking the hormone to help develop breasts and other female physical characteristics call estrogen their "happy
pills." Estrogen elevates mood and adds a glow to life. Estrogen deprivation results in the opposite: feeling down or
emotionally flat.

> "I'm happily married and we don't have to worry about ev-
> ery penny. I really feel that I have nothing to complain
> about, and yet I've been feeling depressed."

> "When I skipped a few periods, I felt much better, but
> when my periods come back again, it seems like whatever
> my body has to do to produce them causes real feelings of
> physical depression."

> "I have these bouts of irritability and depression where I
> feel about to burst into tears every minute and I can't seem
> to rouse myself to do anything."

One study showed that 41 percent of the women hospitalized for depression were admitted on the last premenstrual day or the first day of menstrual flow—the two days
estrogen levels are lowest. Another study done at Yale University found that women who were suicidal during a certain time in their cycle, but not at other times, showed a
decreased blood flow to their frontal lobes on those days.
If they were given estrogen, which is a vasodilator, the
blood flow to the frontal lobes increased, and the tendency
toward suicidal thoughts went down.

Some people say that The Pause does not *cause* personality changes, it merely exaggerates existing tendencies.
But even an exaggeration of tendencies is a real problem.
It is the difference between getting angry when appropriately provoked and expressing the same angry response to
a lesser offense, the difference between feeling somewhat

anxious and being incapacitated by anxiety. The basis is physiological, a change in hormonal balance, rather than psychological, something that can be resolved through self-examination and understanding. And these emotional upheavals can go on for months, sometimes even years.

If you do not know that depression or irritability or even rage can be caused by your changing hormones, you are apt to be much harder on yourself.

> "Since my doctor told me that the only symptom of menopause was the change in my periods and that my mood was not related, I began to think that I was simply not a very nice person and I really got down on myself."

If your friends are not voicing similar complaints, you may worry that psychological inadequacies are at the root of your difficulties.

> "I'm really ashamed that I'm having such a hard time with menopause. Maybe if I were emotionally healthier, I wouldn't have these problems."

> "Menopause humbled me. I thought women who complained about menopause were plain weak. I expected to sail right through. I couldn't believe it when I got hit with mood swings, headaches, and hot flashes. I'll tell you, it's sure made me a lot more compassionate toward other women."

You may worry that you are going crazy or may seek psychotherapy without results. According to Dr. John Arpels, "I can't tell you how many women I've gotten off of Prozac, which their internists prescribed for midlife crisis, when what they were experiencing was really an estrogen phenomenon. Most physicians just don't understand this at all."

In my own psychotherapy practice, I have worked with

women for whom the basis of their anxiety and depression was clearly physiological. There was nothing in their life circumstances that could have accounted for it.

EXTREME REACTIONS—AND SOME SOLUTIONS

Extreme emotional reactions can occur as estrogen levels decrease. In fact, 15 to 20 percent of women have periods of *serious* emotional upheaval during The Pause. They may feel that they are going crazy—so anxious they are afraid to leave the house, so angry they cannot control their tempers, so depressed they can't get out of bed.

"Right now, I'm just trying to get up the courage to go to the market. Everything is such a big deal because I don't know how to handle it. I feel like I'm more a child than my children. I can never tell whether I'm going to be able to cope or not."

"Between ages forty-five and forty-eight I would have what I thought were clinically psychotic experiences, even though I'm normally an even-tempered person. I would have moments of rage and moments of depression or despair even though, upon examination, everything seemed to be fine. I couldn't figure out why I wanted to pick up the piano and throw it through the window. I couldn't figure out why I had images of hanging myself from the balcony. I never knew when it would happen so I couldn't make plans to be with people. It was like a bad drug trip. It felt chemically induced and I had no choice but to ride it out."

"I walked into the house after work a few weeks ago and Brad and the kids were eating dinner. When I saw every cupboard and drawer was open, I started shrieking at them. The intensity of my rage was unbelievable. But at the same time that I was raging, another part of me was saying, 'What are you doing? Stop this! This is really crazy behavior.' But I had absolutely no control. Even though I knew it was inappropriate, I couldn't stop it."

"This is much stronger than PMS and comes in the most unpredictable ways. PMS never defeated me. But now I find myself curled up in a ball on the bed and I just want to die. I want to be left alone and never see anyone again. With PMS I wouldn't allow myself to do this. I'd tell myself that this was just my body and it isn't really how I feel and it will go away in a little while. But this is so open-ended. It seems to go on and on for days and weeks and it's much more intense. It's worn me down and it's frightening me."

According to Dr. Ricardo J. Fernandez, a Princeton, New Jersey, psychiatrist who specializes in hormonally induced depressions, "Emotional illness can definitely be symptomatic of a physical disorder, but most physicians do not realize that. Unless a woman shows classic physical symptoms that would warrant hormonal treatment, physicians tend not to recognize depression as a true medical disorder and often refer the patient to a psychiatrist. One woman I saw was feeling suicidal because her irritability and mood swings were getting so bad. Since she had a prior psychiatric history, her gynecologist felt it was psychiatric rather than hormonal or medical. I did some testing and found her FSH and LH were quite elevated. I started her on estrogen and she improved remarkably over the next few weeks."

There are those who, in an attempt to emphasize the fundamental equality of the sexes, would minimize the effects of hormones upon our emotional equilibrium, and at times the feminist in me is tempted to say that in this regard we are no different from men. But in truth we are. And while many women remain emotionally unaffected by the change in their hormonal balance, others *are* affected to varying degrees. Certainly this does not mean that we are rendered incompetent at this time in our lives, and denying us opportunities because of potential vulnerability to hormone fluctuations is unwise, unfair, and unjust. In fact, whenever I think about this, I am reminded of a radio program I did with Dr. Sadja Greenwood, author of *Menopause Naturally*. A man called in and said it was precisely this reason that a woman should never be elected president. "How could we honestly believe that she could handle the nuclear war 'button' if her hormones were in flux?" he demanded. To this the incensed Dr. Greenwood replied, "There is no question that raging hormones are a problem. It has been the raging of the male hormone, testosterone, that has been responsible for war and devastation over the centuries. I'll take my chances with a menopausal woman anytime."

However, the fact that we do have fluctuations means that women need to know that this transition can produce temporary emotional disequilibrium, but that there are solutions that can help to stabilize or even completely eliminate these unpleasant consequences.

Hormones

For women who have extreme emotional reactions to The Pause, estrogen can be a real blessing. And you do not have to wait until after you have had your last period to benefit—as most doctors generally advise. Since emotional instability either before your period or throughout the month can be caused by estrogen dropping below its set-point, you may find that taking small doses of estrogen during the time in your cycle when symptoms generally appear can even out your emotions.

* * *

"I was getting so angry and frustrated. I would be driving and the car in front of me wouldn't be going fast enough. If I couldn't get around it, I would have fantasies of machine-gunning out the tires. It was like I was inhabited by this other crazy person. I may not be the most mellow person in the world, but I'm not rageful either. Finally, I went on hormones, but the first dose was so low that it didn't do anything. Eventually, I got a dose that worked and my feelings evened out."

"The important thing is to begin with a low dose of estrogen and work up," advises Dr. Roger Lobo, professor of gynecology at the University of Southern California. "If women get too much estrogen, it raises their set-point. Then it becomes a real problem if they want to reduce the dose. Every little drop precipitates symptoms and you get into a sort of roller coaster, requiring higher and higher doses of estrogen because of the new set-point that has been established."

Although several studies show an increase in enhanced mood for women taking estrogen, it doesn't work for all women. It is very successful for minor depression, but the low doses of estrogen generally prescribed for menopausal symptoms are not effective for many cases of serious depression. And some small percentage of women find that the estrogen actually *causes* negative emotional reactions.

"I couldn't take estrogen. I tried Premarin and the patch, and with both of them I was so depressed and so angry all the time that I just couldn't live with myself."

Sometimes these negative reactions occur because the kind of estrogen being used (Premarin is generally less effective than Estrace for minor depression), or the dose taken, is not correct for the particular woman.

While synthetic progesterone frequently has a negative effect on emotional mood, natural progesterone in capsule, cream, oil or sublingual form effectively alleviates premenstrual symptoms for some women.

Herbs

Vitex, or chasteberry, is an herb that appears to balance female hormones. According to Anna Harvey, a chiropractor and medical herbalist practicing in Northern California, "Vitex seems to affect the pituitary. Consequently, it seems to work for women whose estrogen is high as well as for women whose progesterone is high. It works for PMS symptoms as well as menopause symptoms. You can make a tea of the dried berries or take it in tincture form. It is a very gentle, but slow-acting herb. Unfortunately, it can take two to three months before you notice its effects."

"I took chasteberry because I was having horrible emotional swings. Some little thing would happen but it felt like the end of the world. After taking chasteberry for a couple of months, I felt better. But I got lazy and didn't take it all the time. When I stopped taking it, some of the emotional sensitivity returned. It indicated to me that the herb was helping, so I'm taking it regularly now."

A tea made of the herb skullcap can also be useful when you feel irritable, edgy, or anxious. Saint-John's-wort can be used for hormonal or chemical depression, but not for depressions caused by life circumstances.

Acupuncture and Chinese Herbs

Acupuncture and Chinese herbs work for a lot of women. In Chinese medicine, feelings of irritability are considered to be manifestations of a liver disturbance. There are a number of Chinese herbal formulas, available through most acupuncturists and herbalists, that deal with this problem.

"I was very irritable and moody and anxious. Then I had acupuncture and took two Chinese herbal remedies: Two Immortals and Quiet Contemplative, and that evened me out."

Homeopathy

Some women reported that homeopathy helped their emotional swings.

"Within two days of taking the homeopathic Female Glandular formula, I felt like a veil had lifted. For several days I almost felt euphoric. I thought, 'This isn't so bad; I can cope with this.' I was in control of my temper. When midcycle arrived, some of the irritability came back, but it wasn't as bad as before and my breasts were less tender."

Vitamins and Diet

In mild to moderate cases, vitamin B-6 may help reduce the emotional symptoms of PMS. Start with 50 milligrams of B-6 twice a day, and work up to no more than a total of 300 milligrams daily. Time-release tablets are best. (Optivite, Rejuvex, Pro-Woman, and de Buren's Optimum International, Inc., have special hypoallergenic PMS vitamin formulas that are high in B-6.)

Be careful to stay under 300 milligrams per day of B-6 because it can cause serious neurological problems in high doses. You will feel a tingling and numbness in your fingers and toes if you take too much. Natural sources of vitamin

B-6 are chicken, fish, pork, eggs, unmilled rice, soybeans, oats, whole wheat, peanuts, and walnuts.

If you feel emotionally unstable, cut out alcohol and caffeine; they cause estrogen to be flushed out of the body through the urine.

Cut down on sugar. Increased sugar causes high levels of blood sugar which then drop precipitously, often causing or exacerbating negative mental and emotional reactions.

Instead of sugar, eat complex carbohydrates (starchy vegetables, dried beans, peas, pasta, and grains) to keep your blood sugar more even. This doesn't mean you can't cheat on occasion, but the more you keep off sugar, particularly in the second half of the cycle, the fewer symptoms you are likely to experience. Eating small meals throughout the day will also help keep your blood sugar levels more constant.

"My mood swings seem to be highly correlated with blood sugar. I find that if I have four or five small meals a day, I feel better. If I let my blood sugar go down I get catapulted into a real emotional state."

Increase your magnesium to help control PMS symptoms. A lack of magnesium causes a specific depletion of brain dopamine, resulting in anxiety, irritability, and nervous tension. Diets high in vegetables and unrefined grains are much higher in magnesium than diets that include large quantities of refined foods, meat, and dairy products.

Also, calcium and magnesium need to be balanced: three parts calcium to one part magnesium. If you ingest too much calcium in proportion to magnesium, you are more likely to have or aggravate PMS symptoms. If you have a high sugar intake and/or a high calcium intake, you'll want to take extra magnesium in tablet form, 150 to

400 milligrams per day. (If you take too much magnesium, you will get diarrhea.)

Decrease dairy products. Dairy products also deplete magnesium. According to one study, a combined excessive intake of dairy products and sugar can result in chronic magnesium deficiency.

Cut down your intake of salt. Salt increases water retention and the feeling of bloatedness. If you are retaining water, instead of taking a diuretic which can create chemical imbalances in the body (particularly by depleting potassium), increase your water intake and lie down for a while with your feet elevated. This creates better blood flow to the kidneys and allows you to excrete the extra water by urinating.

Finally, don't smoke. Smoking exacerbates every symptom and problem that can accompany menopause.

To minimize PMS symptoms:

Increase	*Reduce*
Vitamin B-6 (50–300 milligrams per day)	Processed foods
	Dairy products
Magnesium (150–400 milligrams per day)	Caffeine
	Alcohol
Whole natural foods (fruits, vegetables, grains)	Sugar
	Salt

Exercise

Exercise regularly, especially when you are feeling out of sorts. Exercise increases brain endorphins, blood flow, and oxygen in the cells—all of which can make you feel better.

One study at Kings College Hospital in London showed that women who exercised regularly *before* The Pause were less likely to be depressed during it. Another study from Stockholm, Sweden, found that women who engaged in regular exercise had a significantly lower degree of meno-pausal symptoms, including less negative mood, when compared with women who did not exercise.

> "Exercise is the only dependable thing. I actually need ex-ercise more for my emotions than my body. Unfortunately, when I am feeling this way, I don't want to go out and do anything, but I force myself because I know that if I get out there, I can run it off."

Exercising relaxes you and reduces stress. And if you are more relaxed and less stressed, your relationships with oth-ers are bound to be more pleasant. "Now that Maggie is exercising and eating well," reported one woman's partner, "she is less stressed and we are getting along a lot better."

Identification and Relaxation

Even though you may feel out of control, you may find you have more control over your emotions once you begin to pay attention to your feelings in a different way. Begin by looking for signs of agitation, irritation, or emotional upset while they are still small. Then see whether a prob-able cause for the feelings comes to mind. Your responses may seem emotionally based, but they may not be.

Question your feelings, and if you cannot easily see a concrete cause for them, take a deep breath, and relabel the feelings as a symptom of hormonal imbalance that re-quires respectful and tender handling. I find that when women can label their reactions as something caused by The Pause, they are often able to manage the emotional upheavals more easily.

"I figure when I don't like how loud my husband breathes, there is something going on in *me* and not *him*. Or he's standing there reading the mail and it bugs me because I want him to be doing something else. Then I say, 'Okay, Lydia, something is going on with you,' and that helps me distance from the intensity of the feelings. I put my feelings in this little box called menopause. And I find I can control it better when I label it and acknowledge it."

"Knowing that it wasn't psychological, that it was simply menopause, made my mood swings easier to manage."

Next, check to make sure you have eaten something recently, since low blood sugar can exacerbate emotional distress.

Then, see whether you can move or postpone your next scheduled activity and take some time to get yourself back into equilibrium. The lost time will be easily regained once you feel better and are more productive.

Walk around the block, take a bath, or close your eyes and either focus on your breathing or imagine yourself in a calm, nurturing, soothing atmosphere. Maybe mentally re-create a past vacation or special experience. Then bask in the calm good feelings for as long as you can. If you lose the image, try to recapture it, or create another.

"Sometimes I'll listen to music or try a little meditation. It makes me feel more relaxed and when I'm more relaxed, I'm less irritable."

"I try not to take things so seriously at this time. I baby myself; maybe I'll take a bubble bath or put on a CD no one else likes to listen to. And I try not to feel guilty when I do things I like."

When you feel short of patience, avoid things that will aggravate you. Postpone that potentially unpleasant encounter for another day. Isolate yourself and work alone if you don't feel fit for human company.

"As soon as I sense this feeling coming on, I go off alone. I won't talk to anyone because I don't want to push this emotional instability onto anyone else."

If you do have to be with people, slow yourself down; take a few deep breaths to soften that edge.

"I try to keep my temper under control. Instead of flying off at people I just try to be as calm as I can. I work to get the irritability out of my voice and talk more calmly."

Another thing you can do is to drop an upsetting issue temporarily while you give yourself time to gain perspective.

"If I find I'm getting angry about something, I let go of it by telling myself that if I'm still angry in two days, I'll deal with it then. In a day or two, the feelings are either gone or they're clarified."

When it comes to human emotions and negotiations, a few hours or even a day rarely matter. What is important, however, is that you find a way to put things in perspective.

Communication

Once you become aware that you are feeling emotionally unbalanced, tell those around you.

"I tell my partner what is happening to me. I'll say something like, 'Sorry I'm in such a bad mood, I don't want to be. I'm not my right self.' "

"Usually I warn my family so they know not to do anything deliberate to irritate me. My teenage son knows this means that he has to get out of my way. If he thinks I'm being unfair, he gets to say it once. Then if he still has feelings, he has to deal with them somewhere else. And I tell my husband the same thing. That way they won't get caught up in my process and it's easier for all of us."

Since these feelings can be so unpredictable and one day can be so different from the next, many partners appreciate a running commentary. So let your partner know how your day is going; how anxious or upset you are feeling; how frequently you are being besieged by hot flashes. It's like a daily weather report: storm brewing or clear skies ahead.

"It's helpful when my wife says to me, 'Look, I'm really not angry with you; I'm having a hard time.' I appreciate it when she says, 'I'm going to rave today. Anyone who comes in the kitchen is likely to get it, so stay out.' I don't like it, but I appreciate it."

Try not to lash out or blame your partner when you feel out of sorts. And, if you do, be certain to apologize. Your partner is likely to be more supportive and forgiving of your emotional upheavals when you take responsibility for your end of the interaction. While you have the right to special concern and thoughtful consideration during this time, you do not have the right to be rude or insolent. Saying that you appreciate your partner's patience and support—in so many words and frequently—will encourage tolerance and compassion.

It is important not only to explain your state of mind to your intimates, but to educate your coworkers as well. Describing the problems that accompany The Pause to your colleagues may be difficult, but is definitely worth the risk. For the most part, women report that when they let their officemates know what is going on they are supportive. They do not assume the woman is incompetent, unreliable, or less able to do her job. Quite to the contrary, we all have periods of disequilibrium—coworkers have children in trouble, go through divorces, deal with ill parents. These periods of disequilibrium, like The Pause, are time-limited. Letting your loved ones and your associates know what is happening enables them to be more sensitive to your needs—or maybe just gives them permission to get out of the way.

"I sat down with my coworker and explained what it is like to be inside my body sometimes. I let him know that if I seem to be having a temper tantrum, he shouldn't personalize it. If the issue is important, I ask if we can postpone discussing it for a day; I don't try to resolve things while I'm in this state of mind."

"Sometimes I feel like I'm going to explode and the classroom is not an appropriate place. So I tell my aide to take over. She knows what's going on. And I walk around the building a few times to try and pull myself together. Many times I've returned to the classroom, but had to walk out a second time."

Finally, keep reminding yourself that The Pause *will* end. Your hormones *will* arrive at a new equilibrium and you *will* recover your emotional equanimity.

"When I was around forty-eight, the roller coaster finally stopped. I had a garden and a lot more compassion for myself. I also had all this extra energy that before I had been devoting to just staying sane. I redecorated the house and did a lot of things I had never done before in my life. I took river and bike trips and became more physically active. I'm actually in better shape now than I was twenty years ago."

In the meantime, if you are seriously bothered by these emotional ups and downs, hormones, homeopathy, acupuncture, and herbs are available. Keep in mind that you are not going crazy; this is a physiological process that is causing a psychological reaction, and an antidepressant or antianxiety drug may not be the answer. Therapy or counseling, however, may help you handle this transition more effectively. One of my patients recently said, "These therapy sessions have helped me put things in perspective. I know I'm not going to let my feelings take me over anymore. I can take a nap, a walk, or do something so I can still keep my plans. I may have some bad days, but I know I can get through it. And I appreciate the good days more."

Remember, most women will *not* be overwhelmed by their emotions. However, some will be. In the rare instance that you feel suicidal or unable to cope, get professional help immediately, even if it means walking into the crisis unit of your local hospital or calling a suicide prevention hot line.

Further Information

TO OBTAIN:

Optivite
found in most pharmacies

Rejuvex
found in most health-food stores

Pro-Woman
(800) KICK-PMS

deBuren's Optimum International
(800) 543-3831

CHAPTER

4

Running Out of Steam

Fatigue is one of the most common companions of The Pause. Literally millions of women in our culture are chronically exhausted by the dual responsibilities of home and job. We are so overextended that exhaustion seems a way of life. But a new level of fatigue frequently accompanies The Pause. And it often comes on suddenly.

"Every time I make my bed, I can only think about getting right back into it."

"I found myself having to sit down three times while doing the dishes the other day. I thought, 'What is this? It's just twelve dishes. What's the matter here?' I was simply weary with fatigue."

"A day or two before my period I get to the point where I feel like I have absolutely no energy. And then it goes away when my period comes."

"About a year ago I was so tired that I would go to bed at eight-thirty and sometimes as early as six-thirty. But since I started taking the estrogen, I don't have to anymore."

"Suddenly, I'll become almost narcoleptic. I have to go to sleep, and I have to go to sleep immediately. And that has been happening more and more frequently."

"Fatigue during the early stages of menopause is due about eighty percent of the time to the insomnia and other sleep disturbances that result from a reduction in estrogen," says Dr. John Arpels. "However, twenty percent of the time it can be due to a drop in testosterone. Testosterone is the hormone that makes you feel energetic and sexually interested. Reduced levels of testosterone are likely when a decrease in sexual desire accompanies the fatigue."

When we are suddenly exhausted beyond reason, with no other symptoms, many of us have no idea what is wrong. One woman I talked to had herself tested for AIDS. This intense level of fatigue during the early stages of The Pause is often responsible for women going from doctor to doctor searching for an answer.

"There was a point there when I said, 'Maybe I'm dying.' So I had my liver checked, colonoscopy, you know, all the things you do to make sure that you don't have some terrible disease. I just felt so tired all the time."

For some women, feeling deenergized comes around the time of ovulation, but for most of us it becomes exaggerated just when we start to menstruate.

"This last period, I just felt totally exhausted for no particular reason. I came home and went to bed at about eight o'clock for two nights in a row. Then, the second day of my period, I was right back to normal."

I can remember taking a ski trip the day I got my period. Two hours after arriving, I had to take a nap. I slept for four hours, something I *never* do. And I wasn't even sleep-deprived. It was the first day of my period compounded by the effects of the altitude. Apparently, altitude sickness becomes exacerbated while women are going through The Pause.

In addition, some women may feel exhausted around their periods because they bleed so heavily.

"When I have heavy periods, I get home from work and have to sleep for an hour or so. I just cannot keep my head up or my eyes open."

With heavy bleeding, fatigue can be an indication that you are anemic, meaning you have less iron than you need.

It is also not uncommon for blood tests to turn up a thyroid deficiency at this point in life.

"I was putting on weight and I was also complaining I was tired all the time. My doctor had never heard me complain about fatigue before, so he ran some tests and discovered I had a thyroid condition."

"It only seems logical that when you have a major change in hormones, the effect will reverberate throughout the body," explains Dr. Ifeoma Ikenze, a San Francisco Bay Area physician and homeopath. "The thyroid is only one of the functions that is frequently affected." Since, as a woman gets older, there is an approximate 10 percent increase in thyroid disease every decade, it is a good idea to get a thyroid stimulating hormone level at menopause and then every five years or so thereafter.

For many women, the extreme feeling of fatigue lifts in

the middle of The Pause, and they enjoy a honeymoon of heightened energy. This can happen for a number of different reasons. In some women, progesterone levels drop and leave the receptors free to utilize the available estrogen. In other women, the response is due to relatively high testosterone levels that can occur during The Pause. This honeymoon, like all honeymoons, ends as estrogen drops further still and yet another episode of disequilibrium sets in. Inevitably, however, menstrual periods stop completely, and once women adapt to this final change, their energies often reassert themselves.

"In my late forties I was having horrendous hot flashes and I was really feeling blah. I felt fat, dumpy and lethargic. But a couple of years ago, after my periods stopped, I went through a real sudden shift. I got reactivated, reenergized, interested in being more physically active. It's been up ever since then."

SLEEP DISTURBANCES

Fatigue also results from sleep deprivation. According to several large surveys, women between the ages of forty-five and fifty report a significant increase in sleep complaints. The most common complaint is waking up in the middle of the night and not being able to get back to sleep.

"I just seem to wake up a lot more during the night and I never did that before."

"I can't sleep at night. I've gone a year without proper sleep. I wake up about six to ten times every night. I'll stay awake from twenty to forty minutes depending on how long it takes to get back to sleep. I'm a wreck because of it."

Our hormone levels *do* affect sleep. A number of different studies have shown that female college students experience sleep disturbances just before and during menstruation, when estrogen levels are lowest. Insomnia, disturbing dreams, and fatigue on waking are the typical sleep-related complaints reported by PMS sufferers.

"Sleep disturbances caused by hormones are different from those of the true insomniac, who falls asleep and then wakes up twenty minutes later and can't get back to sleep again until a few hours before it's time to arise," says San Francisco gynecologist Maida Taylor. "It is also different from the early-morning awakenings of the depressed person, who wakes up earlier than she needs to regardless of how late she's gone to sleep. But a lack of *sustained* sleep is the pattern we see with menopause." Women in The Pause seem to wake up repeatedly during the night because they need to urinate or have had a hot flash or night sweat, or for no apparent reason at all.

"I suddenly start to perspire in the middle of the night. I don't mind the perspiration so much, but it wakes me up and then it's hard to go back to sleep again."

"I often wake up because of really intense hot flashes. Along with the hot flash comes an escalated heartbeat, so I'm breathing hard and my heart is pounding. It's really hard to relax and it can take a long time to go back to sleep."

Regardless of the cause, the result is a lack of continuous, truly restful sleep. In time, such sleep deprivation can wear you down and play havoc with your mood as well as your ability to think clearly.

"I'm so exhausted from lack of sleep that I've sort of lost my objectivity, not to mention my sense of humor. I have this growing fear that it's going to go on forever. I know this is irrational, but I can't see any end. I'm so exhausted that I keep canceling dates and things I really want to do."

Diet, Exercise, and Relaxation

There are some things you can do to help yourself sleep. Cut out caffeinated beverages, including caffeinated soft drinks—if not completely, then certainly after noon. As we age, many of us become more sensitive to stimulants. We also become more sensitive to alcohol, so you may also need to avoid alcoholic beverages in the evening.

Don't eat a large meal just before going to sleep. However, a small bedtime snack can prevent night hunger pangs. Don't drink after dinner if you find you have to wake up to urinate. Sometimes using white noise or playing a recording of the sound of waves crashing or birds singing can help relax you into sleep and prevent noises from jarring you awake.

If hot baths don't induce hot flashes, they may provide a solution to your sleep problems. Dr. Quentin Regestein of the Sleep Clinic at Brigham and Women's Hospital in Boston suggests, "A twenty- to thirty-minute bath, as hot as you can stand it, just before bedtime, raises body temperature. Research shows that raised body temperature leads to deeper sleep. It doesn't work for everyone, and not everyone can tolerate a hot bath comfortably, but if a woman can, it can be a practical and effective treatment." Dr. Regestein continues, "Aerobic exercise sessions, at least thrice weekly for thirty minutes, are another effective means of preventing insomnia. If exercise delays sleep onset, you need to do it earlier in the day."

Relaxation techniques can also get you back to sleep. First, empty your mind of all thoughts and worries. If your mind is in a hyperactive state, if you are working out a problem or you are having some good ideas that you don't

want to forget, write them down. Once they are safely recorded on paper, you may be able to let go of them more
easily. Or, you might just read—something technical or
boring is far better than an engrossing novel, which is
likely to keep you up turning pages.

"My rule of thumb is, if I'm awake for half an hour, I get
up and do something, like read, then I go back to bed."

When you are ready to go back to sleep, close your eyes
and spend a few minutes looking at a black screen in your
mind's eye while listening to your breathing. If a thought
sneaks in, just let go of it by refocusing on the black screen
and the sound of your breathing. Once you can hold a
blank mind for a minute or two, carry out one of the following two simple physical relaxation techniques.

Progressive relaxation, pioneered by Dr. Edmund Jacobson in the early 1960s, involves concentrating on relaxing
your body part by part. Start with your toes, then your
foot, your ankle, your calf, your knee, your thigh—first one
leg, then the other. Progress very slowly up to your head,
body part by body part, until your whole body is relaxed.

The Relaxation Response developed by Dr. Herbert
Benson is a different but equally easy-to-follow relaxation
method. It consists of tensing your entire body all at
once—your hands, arms, legs, feet, stomach, even your
facial muscles. Hold the tension for six seconds, then relax
everything at once, exhaling fully. After ten seconds of relaxation, repeat the process. Two repetitions are generally
sufficient to get you back to sleep within a short while.

Herbs

Natural herbal sedatives are often effective; you can buy them at health-food stores. Ask for passionflower, motherwort, or valerian. They come in capsules or tinctures that can be mixed with water or taken undiluted. Motherwort is particularly appropriate for women in menopause because it also helps balance hormones. You can keep the tincture and a glass of water next to the bed at night. If motherwort is not strong enough, you can use valerian. However, some women report that valerian gives them a druglike hangover. For me, it saved the day—or night— for months. I never went anywhere without my valerian drops. When I had difficulty falling back to sleep, I just took fifteen to thirty drops in water and within fifteen minutes I'd be back off to never-never land. And even if I took it at four in the morning, I'd be fine a few hours later when I awoke.

A good over-the-counter Chinese herbal formula for insomnia is Tian Wan Bu Xin Bang.

Hormones

Estrogen decreases wakefulness and the frequency of awakenings. It cuts down on sleep-disturbing hot flashes and increases REM sleep. REM sleep is the level of sleep that occurs while you are dreaming. A certain amount of REM sleep is essential in order to feel rested and well.

Some researchers postulate that a fall in tryptophan, which is the precursor of serotonin, a neurotransmitter often associated with sleep, is the cause of some sleep disturbances during The Pause. Free plasma tryptophan levels increase when women are treated with estrogen. And many women on sleeping pills are able to get off them once they begin taking hormones. A warm glass of milk before bed increases tryptophan levels as well.

MENTAL FUZZINESS

Even with sufficient sleep, some women going through The Pause complain about a loss of mental acuity, problems with short-term memory, and an inability to concentrate.

"I used to listen to music when I worked. Now I find I have to turn it off at certain times to concentrate."

"I always had a great memory. If someone would say, 'I'll meet you at such and such a place in two weeks,' I'd be there. Now I forget the end of a joke. And sometimes I can't remember words. Last week, I suddenly couldn't remember my best friend's name."

"I don't remember a damned thing. I'm upstairs and I go downstairs. Suddenly I realize I forgot something so I have to go back upstairs to get it. But when I get back up there, I can't remember what the hell I came up for."

My second year into The Pause, I was waiting in the green room to be interviewed on *Oprah*. Ten minutes before we were to go on the air, my period started. During the program I felt as if I were wading through molasses. When I was back home and watched the tape, I was stunned. I missed a number of points I should have made. Two days later I was back in form, but by then millions of viewers had seen me fumble.

Remember that estrogen levels affect the brain, and this will influence mental as well as emotional functioning.

Dr. Bruce McEwen and his colleagues from the Laboratory of Neuroendocrinology at Rockefeller University in

New York have been studying the effect of estrogen on the brains of female rats. "Estrogen definitely affects the number of synapses in the hippocampus in rats," Dr. McEwen told me. "This is a part of the brain that is involved in learning and memory. Lowered estrogen levels mean fewer synapses. While human female brains are quite different from rats', there are some similarities. I would predict from our studies that a decrease in estrogen would cause, in women, some decline of cognitive performance around certain kinds of memory."

I'm usually very efficient at scheduling and organizing my work. But since The Pause, solutions to logistical problems that had always come easily often don't surface until hours later. For example, one day recently, a friend called to change a meeting time. I had to call her back three times before I came up with a viable alternative.

When you can't trust your memory, you have to rely on aids. Women I talked to devised all sorts of fail-safe techniques to augment their capricious memories.

"I have to be much more organized than I used to be. I now write everything down in this book, absolutely everything."

"I carry a little packet of Post-its with me wherever I go. I carry them in my purse, in my pockets, in my car, because I don't trust myself. I now have a place for everything. My keys have a hook, my purse is always on the same shelf, I keep all telephone messages in one book, and I have reading glasses stashed wherever I might need them."

This memory deficit does not affect all women. Some of us make enough estrogen or testosterone to keep our brains going quite well. (The testosterone can either be utilized directly by certain receptors in the brain centers or it can be converted to estrogen and then used by the brain.)

Others of us, however, will have problems. If you believe your ability to understand or react appropriately to new data is being hampered, or if you find that although your memory for historical events remains good, you can't remember that great thought you had five minutes ago, or where you last put your glasses down, additional estrogen may provide the solution.

Recent research by Dr. Barbara Sherwin of McGill University in Montreal shows that estrogen is effective in enhancing several measures of cognitive functioning. "We found that estrogen had a positive effect on short-term memory for women who went through menopause as a result of having had their ovaries removed," Dr. Sherwin reports. "Estrogen also enhanced their ability to learn new material." In general, estradiol has a more positive effect on mental functioning than equine estrogens, like Premarin, because 10–15 percent of the latter does not fit human brain receptors.

In much older age, we see dementia, a severe loss of mental functioning. Apparently the lack of estrogen can play an important role in this deterioration process. Not only do three times as many women suffer from dementia as compared to men, but recent studies show a 93 percent reduction in dementia for women who are currently taking estrogen. And obese women, who naturally manufacture higher levels of estrogen, are *less* likely than thin women to develop this disorder. Research on estrogen and the brain has begun only recently. Within a few years, we should know much more about this important area.

STRESS

Without question, stress affects our menstrual cycles. It is not uncommon to skip a period during final exams, when starting a new job, or after the death of a loved one or some other traumatic event. Stress increases norepinephrine and adrenaline and apparently has a direct biochemical effect on lowering estrogen levels, thereby exacerbating estrogen withdrawal symptoms. And if there is one stressful period of life, it is our forties and early fifties, when many of us have to deal not only with a job and running a household, but with difficult teenagers or ill parents as well.

"The hardest part of my menopause was when my sixteen-year-old stepdaughter was having problems with the law, my mother-in-law was dying, and I was having hot flashes every forty minutes."

With children gone, you may find yourself trying to re-enter the work force or confronting a loveless marriage that was kept together for the sake of the children. While child-rearing may have masked relationship problems, incompatibility, or a lack of intimacy, you may now have to deal with these realities, perhaps facing the possibility of divorce and beginning all over again. Women also tend to marry men who are older, and many face the death of a spouse at this time.

Research has shown that women who experience the greatest number of symptoms during The Pause are those who are married, with children still at home. Single and childless women, who have fewer emotional demands to meet, are likely to fare better (unless, of course, they are recently divorced or widowed). Highly educated women, or those who have a career and enjoy their work, are likely to find the transition easier than those who are less educated and straining to produce an income, working for economic survival rather than personal satisfaction. In every instance, the more stressful the woman's life circumstances, the more difficult her transition through menopause.

It should be mentioned, however, that stress can also produce a powerfully positive impact if handled well. With children gone, you may have more freedom to pursue certain goals, to revitalize relationships, go off on an extensive, non-child-oriented vacation. You may choose to leave a loveless marriage and set off on your own. You may also be discovering the joys of being a grandmother.

When stress does coincide with The Pause, there are things you can do to help manage it and in so doing maintain your homeostasis. The first is to rely on friends for support. Women who have a strong social network have fewer somatic symptoms. The more people you have available as confidants, the more easily you can get through this period.

Relaxation

The best antidote to stress, of course, is rest and relaxation.

> "My feeling is that stress intensifies the physiological reaction. When I'm not under stress, like when we go away for the weekend, my hot flashes, rages, and insomnia are not as intense."

Relaxation exercises such as those I described to help you fall back to sleep can be practiced a couple of times a day during stressful periods. Or you can use a mental imaging or daydreaming technique. "Imaging is the quickest and easiest way to get people to relax," says Dr. Martin L. Rossman, author of *Healing Yourself.* "Just daydream about a peaceful, relaxing place where you enjoy being. Take a few deep breaths, put your shoulders down, and hang out there for three to five minutes, two to four times each day. Soon, you'll begin to feel better. Then you are likely to make more time for this relaxation technique, not because you 'should,' but because it makes you feel good."

Vitamins and Herbs

If you are under a great deal of stress, you may find it helpful to take 50 milligrams of vitamin B complex twice a day. It turns out that when the body's glandular system is overstimulated by stress, the body's resources of vitamin B complex may become depleted. Increasing your vitamin C intake during times of stress can also be helpful. Siberian ginseng in tablets or tinctures or a tea of Siberian ginseng works on the adrenal gland to help your body adapt to stress and restore energy.

Exercise

Hormones, homeopathy, acupuncture, and herbs are all viable approaches to dealing with physical and mental fatigue. But equally important, if not more so, is regular exercise. Exercise relaxes muscles. When you exercise, you use some of that nervous pent-up energy, leaving your body calmer, which makes it easier to sleep. Exercise energizes rather than depletes you. It is also likely to raise your spirits. So even if you don't *feel* like working out, when you do, the endorphins that are released are likely to make you feel better.

"I can be very tired in the morning and I won't want to exercise, but if a friend invites me to play tennis for an hour, I'm so happy I went. I feel so much lighter and relaxed afterward and I sleep better."

So try to exercise daily—twenty minutes out of a day is not a great deal of time. Exercise should be a priority. Schedule your exercise first and then plan the rest of your day around it.

5

Headaches, Hot Flashes, and Other Miseries

Unless a woman has reached her late forties or is into her fifties, most physicians still do not immediately think of the hormonal changes of menopause as an explanation for many vague physiological complaints such as aching joints, frequent urination, headaches, and digestive problems. And while you are unlikely to experience all of the symptoms covered in this chapter, you will probably have a couple of them.

Some of you will experience a number of symptoms, as I did. If this happens, the information provided here will prepare you to help your health practitioner with your diagnosis. It will also provide you with a variety of treatment options. Unless you are armed with information about the possibilities for your own treatment, you are likely to be neglected. With information, you can monitor your progress through The Pause and choose wisely among the options that are open to you.

ACHING JOINTS AND MUSCLES

Joint and muscle aches—backaches, hip pain, cramping of the legs or feet—are common among women navigating The Pause. Sure, it might just be a sign of aging, but lower levels of estrogen *can* reduce muscle strength and increase the experience of stress on your joints as well.

"My wrists and my right thumb were painful at times. Last Thanksgiving, I couldn't clear the dishes away from the table because my wrists were killing me. But since I have gone on hormones, they haven't been bothering me at all."

"I get this pain in my right shoulder. I used to think it was tension from sitting too long. But I just had the shoulder pain a couple of days before my period started. After my period, the pain went away. Now that I look back and think about it, it always starts around that time."

Women of many nationalities experience joint pain during The Pause. Forty percent of Nigerian women complain of joint and bone pain. The most common symptom of menopause in Japan is stiff or sore shoulders. In the Western world, women between the ages of forty and fifty are the most likely group to develop "frozen shoulders," a painful ailment that restricts shoulder motion.

What can you do if you experience muscle or joint discomfort? Exercise strengthens muscles. Massage will help ease the pain. Reduction of pain is one of the best-proven outcomes of acupuncture. Teas made from herbs that cleanse the liver, such as burdock, black cohosh, or blue cohosh, and kidney cleansers, like nettles and cleavers, can reduce joint pain. And estrogen supplementation increases blood flow and oxygen in the cells, and improves the production of joint fluid.

GASTRIC UPSET

Women commonly complain about gastrointestinal upset during The Pause. Not only do they talk about constipation, diarrhea, and indigestion during this time, but many seem to be plagued by flatulence.

> "Another problem for me is gas. My stomach boils. It makes so much noise it could keep you awake at night. I also have this watery, gassy stool and it's real uncomfortable."

> "About a week before my period I get constipated and I have a lot more gas."

There are estrogen receptors in the stomach and small intestine which are affected by changing levels of hormones. A decrease in estrogen causes an increase in hydrochloric acid in the stomach, which can cause stomach upset. Relatively higher progesterone levels relax the intestinal tract. This means waste takes longer to go through the bowel. The result can be constipation and gas. Whether estrogen levels are too low or progesterone is relatively too high, estrogen supplementation should provide help.

In addition to homeopathy and acupuncture, herbs can also be quite effective for minor digestive problems. The Chinese herbal formula Shu Kan Wan counteracts bloating and gas. Chamomile or peppermint tea taken with or after a meal can curtail gas. Eating a bitter herb, such as arugula, turnip greens, or mustard greens, before a meal stimulates digestion. A teaspoon of psyllium husks, found in most health-food stores, can be mixed with a full glass of water to reduce constipation. Many people prefer to mix the psyllium husks with apple juice, creating an applesauce-like mixture.

NAUSEA AND DIZZINESS

Relatively high estrogen levels can lead to nausea either premenstrually or midway through the cycle. Nausea and dizziness may also be due to a relatively higher progesterone level, which can cause an increase in the release of prostaglandins in the secretory lining of the uterus during menstruation. In addition, hot flashes can cause dizziness or a kind of exhaustion that is reminiscent of a low-grade flu.

"I have a lot of trouble with physical balance. I'll notice that I'm off balance every so often. I'll go to put one foot in front of the other or something and I'll feel dizzy."

"Two or three days before I get my period I feel nauseated, especially when I wake up. It's almost like I have a mild stomach virus. I don't feel like throwing up or anything, I just feel queasy until after I've eaten."

During The Pause, some women become more sensitive to changes in altitude and get altitude sickness at high elevations. So when planning that next ski vacation, you might want to schedule sufficient time to relax for a day or two before you head for the slopes.

HEADACHES

Forty percent of American women experience headaches while going through The Pause.

"At forty-three, I started to get a mild headache three days before my period. Since I never get headaches, it was notable. But it wasn't a problem, only a signal that my period was coming."

"I'm not prone to headaches, but when I was thirty-nine, I had a headache that took my breath away. And ever since, I've had monthly headaches that are clearly hormonal. Some months they are gentle, and some months they are fierce, but they come on the dot. When my headache comes, I can tell you when my period will start."

In fact, there is a headache called a "menstrual migraine" that is caused by a lack or sudden withdrawal of estrogen, which can cause constriction of blood vessels going to the brain. It generally starts two or three days before menstruation and goes away one or two days after bleeding begins. The drop in estrogen that occurs just before or at ovulation can also cause headaches.

"For about three to five days right in the middle of my cycle, I get these huge headaches. They are profound. They can go all day and night."

Since a relative excess of progesterone creates the same constriction of blood vessels going to the brain as having too little estrogen, some women experience headaches during the second half of the cycle, when their progesterone levels are too high compared to their estrogen levels.

According to Dr. John Arpels, "If you add small doses of estrogen for just a few days, beginning 24 to 48 hours before the point where the woman expects to get a headache, if she takes estrogen pills or uses the estrogen patch, for example, the cerebral vessels get the estrogen they need so they won't go into spasm and she won't have a headache. If she can't anticipate it, she can take estrogen sublingually at the first sign of a headache."

It is important for women with headaches to keep their estrogen levels constant, but the best way to do this depends on the response of the individual woman. Consequently, Dr. Edward Lichten, director of the Headache

Institute for Women in Southfield, Michigan, uses a variety of approaches. "In my experience, headache patients often do not do well on oral estrogen. This may be due to their extreme sensitivity to estrogen levels because estrogen levels decrease over the 24 hours as the hormone is metabolized. Some of these women do better splitting the pill and taking one-half twice a day. Others do better on the patch which provides a constant flow of hormone; and some women I have treated have done well on injections when they have not responded to anything else."

There are other causes of headaches. Some are prompted by the excessive release of prostaglandins. These headaches start a couple of days before the period and can also be accompanied by bad menstrual cramps and diarrhea. They can be treated by an antiprostaglandin such as Motrin.

While The Pause can *cause* headaches for some women, ironically, *menopause* may solve the problem permanently for others who have been plagued by menstrual migraines for years. With no withdrawal of estrogen each month, their headaches often disappear.

In addition to estrogen supplementation, women I interviewed had successfully alleviated their headaches with alternative therapies including the herb feverfew, homeopathic remedies, acupuncture, and Anacin. One woman touted the benefits of aromatherapy.

"I have cluster headaches, like a girdle centered above my eyes. I get them midcycle. I went to a talk by an American Indian who spoke about using peppermint oil for headaches. So I bought some on the spot. You rub it vigorously into the center of the forehead just below the hairline. If I do this just as the headache first starts, it goes away and doesn't come back again for another month."

BRAIN STATIC

Instead of headaches, some women describe a kind of "static in the brain."

"Sometimes during the night there will be an electrical charge in my head. It feels like a bolt of lightning going through my brain. There is even a sound that goes with it. It will wake me up either before or at the same time that I have a hot flash."

"I get a feeling of static electricity in my head, like my brain is short-circuiting. And I can hear it. It sounds like electricity and it lasts for a couple of seconds. If I'm thinking about anything, it completely breaks off. When I come out of it I feel confused or disoriented for about ten seconds. I couldn't even remember my name once. But then it goes away. At first I was scared, now I just tell myself not to worry, that it will pass."

Experiencing a buzzing in your head can be downright terrifying unless you know that this is another, although fairly uncommon, symptom of changing hormones, and nothing serious or dangerous.

SKIN SENSITIVITIES

Skin sensitivity is a common symptom associated with estrogen deficiency. The technical term is "formication," a sense of tingling or itching as if ants were crawling over your skin. According to Dr. Maida Taylor of San Francisco, "You don't read much about it in textbooks, but patients come in complaining about it all the time. They describe a burning, itching, stinging, or prickly sensation, or simply a hypersensitivity, a sense that any touch is annoying."

"Sometimes I have this feeling of burning all over my skin, like a jellyfish has touched me."

Because the skin feels so sensitive, some women do not want to be touched. The feeling of irritation may interfere with lovemaking and sexual pleasure. In extreme cases, the sensation of clothing on the skin may feel unbearable.

Estrogen supplementation, homeopathy, and acupuncture can all help reduce skin sensitivity.

BREAST TENDERNESS

It is very common for women to experience breast tenderness premenstrually. However, with The Pause, this period of tenderness may lengthen from a few days to a couple of weeks. It may start as early as ovulation, with the surge of estrogen produced in an attempt to stimulate the egg follicles, and may last until after bleeding begins.

In many women, vitamin E works well to relieve breast tenderness. Begin with 100 international units a day and gradually build up until symptoms diminish. However, do not exceed 800 international units per day without medical supervision.

FREQUENT URINATION

As women's hormones begin to change, frequent urination turns out to be a very common experience. I didn't know this and actually thought I had diabetes for a while. I had to get up more than three times a night to urinate. I couldn't imagine how I was able to manufacture all that urine, since I had nothing to drink after 7 P.M.

According to Dr. Richard Schmidt, professor of urology at

the University of California Medical School in San Francisco, "The sacral nerves that control the pelvis and its organs have a high density of estrogen receptors. A flux in hormonal levels may affect the excitability of the nerves and make you feel like you have to urinate more frequently. If your pelvic muscles are also sore due to poor posture or misuse, like runners who get bad knees, problems can eventuate. Frequent urination may be one of them." Also, progesterone can act as a diuretic. Consequently, relatively high levels of progesterone may be responsible when the problem occurs in the second half of the cycle.

If you are experiencing frequent urination, first rule out other medical causes before you blame The Pause. Make sure, for example, that the urination is not a sign of diabetes or a bladder infection. Bladder infections tend to be more common at this time due to reduced estrogen, which lowers the protective acidity level of the vagina. Urinating immediately following sexual intercourse will help reduce bladder infections.

Caffeinated drinks can cause you to urinate frequently, so reduce your consumption of them, even if you have been drinking them for years. You may be more sensitive to them now. Make sure you do not have a high intake of diuretics—of substances like coffee that cause you to release water. And cut out all liquids before going to bed.

For most women, the real problem created by needing to urinate frequently at night is the fatigue and irritability that result from having their sleep constantly disturbed.

URINARY INCONTINENCE

Many women find that they begin developing stress incontinence or urge incontinence early in The Pause. Stress incontinence means that urine leaks out when you cough, sneeze, or laugh. Urge incontinence refers to the inability to hold back the urine when you feel the impending need to urinate. Urinary incontinence afflicts between 6 and 20 percent of people over sixty-five in the United States. Fifty percent of nursing home residents are estimated to have the problem. But it can begin much earlier.

"My period just started to get irregular a few months ago and now I'm having this bladder control problem. If I have to go, I have to go *right then*."

Urinary incontinence can be a major problem. Not only can women experience a loss of urine with sexual intercourse and orgasm, but unless it is cured, you must resort to sanitary napkins or adult diapers. For some women, the problem is so great that they stop socializing out of embarrassment.

Besides genetics and the aging process, the major cause of urinary incontinence probably stems from voiding incorrectly, Dr. Schmidt theorizes. "Women have a tendency to *push* instead of *relaxing* their pelvic muscles with voiding. This stresses the muscles and nerves of the pelvic floor. After many years of this practice, combined with the normal loss of nerve function due to aging, pelvic muscle tone can diminish significantly."

There are other causes of urinary incontinence: pregnancies, childbirth, pelvic surgery. But these may exacerbate problems that originated with poor voiding habits. With good voiding habits they may not be as problematic in and of themselves.

How does The Pause fit in? Since the pelvic nerve that supplies the bladder is rich in estrogen receptors, it is possible that hormonal changes aggravate an already stressed system.

In the late 1940s Dr. Arnold Kegel developed exercises for the pubococcygeal muscle (or PC muscle) to control urinary incontinence. The PC muscle is the one you *squeeze* to *stop* the flow of urine. Locate it by stopping your urine midstream. Don't use your stomach or buttock muscles to do this; you should be able to squeeze this muscle while the rest of your pelvis is entirely relaxed. However, since the muscle covers the entire pelvic floor, surrounding the anal as well as the vaginal opening, you will also feel the squeeze in your anus. If you are not sure you are squeezing the right muscle, put a finger in your anus or your vagina and see whether you can feel the muscle contract around it. Again, make sure you are *not* squeezing other muscles at the same time.

The following Kegel exercises are reported to significantly reduce stress incontinence in 50 to 90 percent of female patients.

Exercise 1: Squeeze and release the PC muscle ten times slowly. For healthy bladder control, the releasing or relaxing of the PC muscle is just as important as, perhaps even more important than, the tensing. By doing this, you are not simply strengthening the muscles; you are making the function of the muscles more efficient. So don't just concentrate on squeezing, also focus on relaxing the muscle fully.

Exercise 2: Do a series of ten rapid contractions and releases.

Complete the ten contractions for each exercise at *five* different times during the day. Increase the number of contractions until you can accomplish fifteen to twenty squeezes and releases with each exercise. Some women notice a difference after practicing the exercises for a few weeks; others require months. An added benefit of doing the Kegel exercises is that some women observe an increase in pleasure during sexual intercourse.

"There was a period there where I was peeing twenty times a day and a half dozen times at night as well. Also, when I

had coughing or sneezing fits, I would have to wear a sanitary napkin. After I started doing Kegel exercises, I sensed
an improvement. I do them every day—when I answer the
phone and as soon as I get in the car."

For continued bladder health, you should carry out the
Kegel exercises daily for the rest of your life. If you are not
sure you have isolated the correct muscle, you might benefit from biofeedback. A perineometer is a machine that
measures your muscle contractions. A probe is put into the
vagina and the pointer on the perineometer moves when
you squeeze the correct muscle. Research conducted by
the Gerontology Research Center in Maryland showed
that biofeedback was 50 percent more effective than verbal
instructions alone in teaching women to squeeze and relax
the PC muscle.

If you cannot develop efficient control of the pelvic muscles with the Kegel exercises, there are a number of direct
nerve stimulation devices that can be very effective. For
example, a vaginal plug is a device shaped like a tampon
which when inserted into the vagina automatically stimulates these muscles. A physician with a special interest in
incontinence can advise you further about these solutions.

Estrogen cream or hormone replacement therapy may
help resolve mild cases of urinary incontinence. Surgery is
needed in more extreme cases, but still may not work unless you also change your pattern of voiding.

Take the time to teach your children how to relax and
void properly, especially your daughters. Urinary incontinence is a major problem among aging populations in all
Western cultures. In Third World cultures, where there is
less pressure to do everything quickly, including urinating,
incontinence is rare.

ORAL SYMPTOMS AND ODOR

Like the mucous membranes of the vagina, those of the mouth, nostrils and eyes may undergo changes due to the lack of estrogen. Some women experience a dryness or burning sensation in their mouths, a bitter taste, or bad breath. The membranes of the nostrils may also lose moisture and feel drier. Dry eye conditions may result and contact lens wearers may start to develop calcium deposits on their lenses. It is not uncommon to develop underarm or vaginal odors as well.

> "At first I woke up with a distinctive sour taste in my mouth. Then I noticed it was there most of the day. It didn't really bother me except for the fact I knew it was there."

> "My body odor was horrible. By the end of the day I could hardly stand myself and I'd have to go in and take a shower."

During The Pause and particularly postmenopausally, vaginal infections tend to increase. This can account for vaginal odors. As estrogen declines, the vagina becomes less acidic and the lining becomes thinner and more fragile. This means the vagina can get irritated more easily, resulting in more frequent vaginal infections, and occasionally yeast infections. Wearing cotton underwear and vaginally inserting yogurt or acidophilus suppositories, found in most health-food stores, can help prevent yeast infections.

One study at McGill University in Montreal showed that Replens vaginal suppositories, used two to three times a week, were very helpful in restoring the proper acid balance. Also, 15 milligrams of zinc can be taken daily as a prophylactic. Don't douche—douches simply wash away natural secretions and leave the vagina drier and more susceptible to infection.

HOT FLASHES

Hot flashes are the hallmark of menopause. It is estimated that between 75 and 85 percent of American women experience hot flashes during The Pause. For most women, hot flashes will be mild, but 10 percent will be so incapacitated by them that they will seek treatment. Some women begin experiencing hot flashes a number of years before their last period, and some do not have any until after their periods have completely stopped.

Hot flashes validate what may have thus far been only vague and nonspecific symptoms. One woman who was so irritable that she could barely stand herself told me that she wished she would have a hot flash to prove that the irritability was because of The Pause and not some psychiatric problem.

Especially in the early stages of The Pause, some women experience a subtle change in general body temperature rather than full-blown hot flashes.

"I've noticed that it doesn't take much for me to get overheated. When I work out for an hour, I don't get heavy sweats, but I notice this undercurrent of heat within my body that didn't used to be there."

"I was in my late thirties or so when my body temperature began to change a little. I wouldn't get as cold as I used to get. In fact, when normally I would be the one who would want to get another blanket, I was actually removing a blanket. I would get too hot when my husband would cuddle up to me, whereas before I loved it because he kept me warm."

So far, I've only had a few spells of feeling slightly warmed from the inside out. But I'm no longer freezing all the time. I used to be so cold that I'd wear silk underwear if the temperature dropped below sixty-two degrees. Then one day I noticed that I was too warm in my silk underwear and felt comfortable walking around without a jacket, even at a temperature at which I would normally have been shivering. I felt the way I had in my ninth month of pregnancy, pleasantly comfortable.

Initial hot flashes tend to be mild, and some women never experience more than a wave of warmth over their body.

"I have these warm flushes once or twice a day, but they are so light, I hardly notice them. It's this nice little warm toasty feeling that goes out to my fingertips."

"A couple of times a day, mostly when I go into a warm room or bus, my face will get warm and I'll have to shut off the heat or open the windows. It lasts for about ten minutes and then goes away."

"I'll be sweeping or folding laundry or doing something physical and suddenly I'll think 'God, I'm so hot.' So it gets my attention and interrupts what I'm doing. But if I sit down and relax, the heat goes away."

"In the beginning hot flashes were very hard to identify. I would think, that's interesting, maybe I have a little touch of the flu or something, maybe a low-grade fever. So I'd take my temperature, but I didn't have one. When they came in full force they had a definite beginning and definite end, but in the beginning they didn't."

For some women, hot flashes are the torment of The Pause.

"They were so intense and severe that I couldn't concentrate at work. I'm a psychotherapist and I remember one patient talking about just becoming aware that she had been sexually abused as a child. She was in a lot of pain talking about this, but all I could think of was how I could get my clothes off. That was the day I called and asked my doctor to write me a prescription for hormones."

"It feels like an iron has been laid on my clothing and the clothing has been laid against my back. It's awful."

"Once I was having sex with my husband and I thought I was going to burn up from the inside out. I literally expected to see ashes on the bed."

"To call it a hot flash is one thing, but it feels more like a panic attack to me. My heart will race and I'll start to sweat. That's the reaction you have when you're responding to terror. Like, if a rattlesnake appeared on the deck, my physiological experience would make sense, but without it, it's hard to figure out what's wrong."

While complex theories about hot flashes abound, no one yet knows for certain what causes something to go haywire in the hypothalamus, the temperature-regulating part of the brain. For some reason, blood vessels constrict, which increases body temperature. In fact, body temperature can actually rise a few degrees.

"It feels like I'm a heater, that I'm producing heat that radiates all over my body. I get so hot, so intense, that my husband can feel the heat on his side of the bed. He can tell I'm having a hot flash without even touching me."

Within a short time, the body recognizes that it is overheating and you begin to sweat in an attempt to cool off.

"I would feel extremely hot with no way to cool down. Then I'd be soaking wet. It would be like having a high fever. When it breaks and you sweat, it's almost a relief."

Sometimes the sweating leads from feeling overheated to feeling chilled within seconds. These abrupt shifts from one extreme to the other can be quite unsettling.

"My body temperature was either hot or cold at all times. I was never comfortable."

Women can perspire so intensely that the perspiration drips off their faces. When one lawyer soaked her blouse during a hot flash, she had to run out between appointments to buy a new one.

A hot flush—where the coloration of the skin on the chest, neck, or face ranges from light pink to dark red—sometimes accompanies the hot flash. When hot flashes occur at night they are called night sweats.

"I would have night sweats in my thirties and forties. I would wake up and be totally saturated and hot, but this would happen only once a night and not every night so I never gave it much thought."

Before I realized I was experiencing symptoms of The Pause, I remember waking up once or twice a night with perspiration on my forehead, chest, and especially at the nape of my neck. For me, these mild sweats were never uncomfortable. In fact, I missed them when they stopped. However, my experience is not typical. Most women who have night sweats are awakened a number of times at night. They are constantly pulling the covers on or off. Some soak the bed so thoroughly that they have to change the sheets or their nightclothes—one or more times a night. Often they can't fall back to sleep afterward.

"I have those horrible night sweats you hear about. My nightgown gets soaking wet. I have to take my clothes off, take the covers off and lie next to an open window. I feel like I'm bursting. I just lie there for five minutes with no covers. Then I get cold because of the sweat drying so I go under the cover to warm up. And just when I'm getting comfortable, it starts all over again."

Some women experience hot flashes during the day, while others have them only at night. Still others have the great misfortune to be visited by them both day and night. Some have a hot flash once a week or less frequently. My mother had only a few during her entire menopause, and some women never have one. But close to half of us will have them every day, at least for a while, and for some, these hot flashes will be severely incapacitating.

"When they started out, they were very irregular. Then they would come once an hour like clockwork. I thought I was counting contractions. They were one and a half minutes from beginning to end. They would start off with a feeling of achiness and a little warmth and would develop to where I'd want to stand with no body parts touching. After they reached a peak, I would break out in a sweat and it would be over. It got so that I had to wait for the hot flash before I would begin making love. It was only then that I felt I might have some time free from them to enjoy myself."

"For almost a year, I had three to four hot flashes an hour at night and some during the day as well. I just tried to sleep when I could and I guess I got used to it. Every once in a while, I didn't have one. It was like when the baby slept through the whole night the first time: I was ecstatic. I finally went on hormones when I was forty-six and that stopped them."

"It was like three thousand degrees at least twenty times a day and they kept me awake at night. The only time I didn't get them was when I was cold. If I were standing outside without a sweater, I was okay."

For most women, hot flashes last a year or two, but about 25 percent find they last for more than five years, and a few continue to have them sporadically for decades. Hot flashes tend to be worst just around the time when menstrual cycling stops.

> "Before my periods stopped, they weren't that bad, but *after* my periods stopped, they became worse. Every night, and during the day too. No matter where I was, I was wringing wet."

> "I started getting hot flashes about two years before my last period, but they got really bad after menstruation stopped."

If you do continue to get hot flashes, it probably means that your ovaries are still kicking on and off.

> "My periods stopped and I got these incredible hot flashes for four or five months. Then they stopped. Then my periods came back again and the hot flashes returned."

> "I'll have hot flashes for about three to four months and then they'll go away for two to three months. Then just when I get comfortable and think it's all over, they come back. It's like big waves."

Even though such a high percentage of American women experience hot flashes, the phenomenon is by no means universal. For example, only 15 percent of Japanese women have hot flashes. In fact, it is so uncommon in Japan that there is no Japanese word for it. Only 30 percent of Nigerian women report having hot flashes. Hot flashes appear to be prevalent among more Western-acculturated city-dwellers. Unfortunately, we don't know how much of this discrepancy is due to genetics, diet, stress, or environmental factors.

To help control your hot flashes, notice whether anything you do either makes them worse or relieves them. Keep a journal and you may notice some interesting patterns. For example, we know that stress affects hot flashes. A Canadian study demonstrated that when stress was induced in a laboratory setting the frequency of hot flashes increased. When one woman learned that stress could bring on a hot flash, she decided to experiment.

> "Sure enough, I was able to create a hot flash if I thought of something aggravating. So I figured that if I had the control to bring them on, then I had the control to stop them. But no way, not a chance. Nothing I did could turn them off."

While mind control may not work, there *are* things you can do to eliminate hot flashes—or at least make them more bearable.

Exercise

Exercise reduces hot flashes. The one study that looked at aerobic conditioning and hot flashes actually showed a significant increase in estrogen levels after exercising. And 55 percent of the women in this study also reported a decrease in the severity of their hot flashes.

> "If I let a day or two go by and I don't exercise, the hot flashes come back much more regularly. I must get them twenty times a day. But when I exercise, I get them maybe half that amount."

Deeper breathing patterns often occur with exercise, and rate and depth of breathing appear to be important factors in controlling hot flashes. A recent biofeedback study showed that women trained to slow and deepen their abdominal breathing pattern showed a 50 percent decline in hot flashes, whereas women who used biofeedback techniques to relax or control alpha waves showed no improvement.

Diet

Avoid coffee, chocolate, alcohol, and spicy foods. Some women react to the acid in such fruits as grapefruits and oranges, tomatoes, and berries, so eat these in combination with other foods.

Eat small meals. Large meals dilate blood vessels and cause the body to grow warmer. Finally, if you are thin, you may want to consider gaining a few pounds. Very thin women have a harder time with hot flashes because they have fewer fat cells for producing estrogen.

Clothing

Natural fibers breathe better. Wear cotton underwear and outer garments of cotton, rayon, and silk. Loose-fitting clothing is generally more comfortable. Especially avoid turtlenecks or anything tight-fitting around the neck. Dress in layers so that you can easily take things off and put them on again. You also may want to cut down on your use of perfume, as hot flashes can make you more sensitive to odors.

At Night

Open the window and turn off the heat when you go to sleep. Keep an ice pack by the side of the bed. Use 100 percent cotton sheets. Sometimes it is easier to sleep in cotton nightclothes that can be changed easily than to sleep nude and have to change the bedding.

"I started wearing long cotton T-shirts to bed. If you had to keep changing sheets on a water bed, you'd find another solution too."

One woman got a king-sized bed because the heat from her husband's body touching her at night would set off a hot flash.

A fan by the side of the bed can be very helpful. A friend of mine installed a ceiling fan with remote control.

"I love the ceiling fan. I rip off the covers and flick the switch and I feel great. The only problem is that my lover hates it because she wakes up with her ears pinned back against her head."

Hints

- Keep a thermos of ice-cold water nearby day and night.
- Take a cold drink at the first sign of a hot flash.
- Try to work by a window or in a well-ventilated area.
- Arrive at meetings early so that you can get the coolest seat.
- Purchase a small portable battery-operated fan (some are purse size), or carry an old-fashioned folding fan.
- Use your freezer liberally. A number of women talked about opening the freezer at home (or in the market) and sticking their head in when a hot flash hit.

"I spent a lot of time with my head resting on the chopped spinach in my freezer. Why the spinach? Because it's not as lumpy as peas or carrots."

- Maintain a regular and active sex life. A Stanford research study showed that women who have inter-

course regularly, one or more times a week, have
fewer or less intense hot flashes.
- Visualization can help. When you have a hot flash,
close your eyes and imagine the heat rushing out
through your hands and feet as you exhale, and
cool air filling your body as you inhale. Or pick
some other cooling image that works for you.

"I try to visualize the heat going through my body and
coming out through my toes. So I sleep with one foot outside the covers. In my image, the heat trails out off my foot
and down to the floor."

Vitamin Supplements

Vitamin E seems to help hot flashes. However, do not
take vitamin E if you have high blood pressure, diabetes,
or a rheumatic heart condition. Start with 100 units for a
few days, then gradually build up until you reach a level at
which the hot flashes diminish. You can take 600 to 800
international units a day without a doctor's supervision.

"I take five hundred units of vitamin E every day faithfully
because it helps my hot flashes. It took a while to kick in,
but after a couple of weeks I definitely noticed a difference."

In high doses vitamin E may be toxic, so stay within the
safe limits. If you experience blurred vision, stop taking it
immediately. Excellent food sources of vitamin E are peanuts, soybeans, spinach, wheat germ, and vegetable oils.
Recently, the bioflavonoid hesperidin has been shown to
alleviate hot flashes when 1,000 milligrams a day is taken.
Bioflavonoids work synergistically with vitamin C, which
helps to strengthen capillaries and regulate body temperature, so take 500 to 1,000 milligrams of vitamin C three
times a day along with the 1,000 milligrams of hesperidin.

Herbs, Acupuncture, and Homeopathy

Siberian ginseng and chasteberry (Vitex) are effective at reducing hot flashes, but they may take a few months before they begin to work. Black cohosh is also effective when used with chasteberry. Dong Quai is another herb that quiets hot flashes.

Homeopathic remedies and Chinese herbal formulas (such as Zhi Bai Ba Wei Wan or Ba Wei Di Huang Wan) can ease hot flashes as well. One Swedish study showed a significant decrease in hot flashes among women who received electro-stimulated acupuncture.

"I'm taking Sepia and a homeopathic female glandular formula and I have fewer hot flashes now."

"I was having very frequent hot flashes. I went to my acupuncturist and he helped me. I was treated with needles and herbs. I did them together, so I don't know which one worked. But it did work."

Hormones

Estrogen is particularly effective at stopping hot flashes. However, should you decide to stop taking the estrogen at some later date, your body will still have to readjust to the decrease in estrogen levels and you are likely to experience hot flashes at that time, so you need to go off the estrogen very gradually. Of course, you can choose to continue to take estrogen throughout your life, but more about that in Chapter 8.

Oral progestins, which are synthetic progesterones such as Provera, stop hot flashes in about half the women and are options for those who cannot take estrogen. However, taking a progestin alone can cause thinning of vaginal tissues, which can mean pain with intercourse. (Pages

123–26 offer an array of solutions for painful intercourse.) Natural progesterone in capsules, cream, oil and sublingual preparations are also often effective for relieving hot flashes. Clonidine and Aldomet are nonhormonal prescription drugs that may be used by women who cannot take estrogen.

There are other conditions besides The Pause that can cause hot flashes and night sweats. They can be symptoms of emotional upset, an overactive thyroid, or high blood pressure that is out of control. Therefore, you should have a medical examination if you are not positive that your hot flashes are being caused by The Pause.

PALPITATIONS

There is nothing scarier than suddenly becoming aware that your heart is racing or beating irregularly for no apparent reason.

> "I often feel like I'm going onstage to speak to fifty thousand people. My heart is racing and I keep looking at my hands because I expect them to be shaking, but they aren't."

Most women who have palpitations experience them while they are having a hot flash. Some have described this combination as something akin to a panic attack. For myself, I experienced these periods of very strong and irregular heartbeats just after I lay down to sleep. I had no hot flashes, but suddenly my heart began to beat thunderously in the quiet of my bedroom. I would change my position in hopes of calming the runaway beast, and this usually helped. But before I knew that palpitations commonly accompanied The Pause, I was petrified.

It appears that heart palpitations are caused by the same vasomotor irregularity that causes hot flashes. In addition, severe angina and chest pain can be experienced by otherwise perfectly healthy women with normal hearts when drops in estrogen cause spasms of the coronary arteries in the same way they cause spasms of the blood vessels to the brain that result in headaches. But since irregular heartbeat and chest pain can be symptoms of a serious heart or circulatory system problem, you may want to get them checked out before chalking it up to The Pause.

When your heart begins beating wildly, try to relax, change your physical position, and breathe deeply. Calm yourself with words of comfort, "This is only a sign of menopause. It is not harmful to my health. In a few moments it will go away." Estrogen supplementation, homeopathy, and acupuncture all address this symptom.

CHANGING PERIODS

If you have a uterus, you cannot enter The Pause without experiencing a change in your menstrual pattern. Even if you have no other symptoms, you will have this one. And while some women simply stop bleeding abruptly one day, irregular bleeding over an extended time is the more common pattern. The Pause can produce a lighter flow or a near-hemorrhage, shorter cycles or longer ones. In fact, a negative response on a pregnancy test after a missed period can be a woman's first awareness that she is entering The Pause.

> "At first, I went from a very reliable, consistent twenty-eight-day cycle to periods that would come in twenty-five days or thirty days."

"I had irregular periods for two years—very irregular. Sometimes there were only three weeks between periods. And I would have these very heavy periods, lasting sometimes ten or twelve days, so I felt like I was bleeding all the time."

"I would miss a period and then they would come every two weeks. My cycle was completely out of whack. I never knew when I was going to have a period and I used to be quite reliable. And now when it comes, the cramping is a lot worse."

"At first, my periods were still regular, but much heavier. I had to change a Tampax every hour. Then, after about six months, it just kind of went back to normal for a while. Then my periods got shorter. They would last for five days instead of the usual seven."

"I had changes in my periods as early as forty-two or forty-three. They became heavier and the consistency was thicker. They also came closer together."

EXCESSIVE BLEEDING

While irregular cycles can go on for years, one of the biggest problems for women can be excessive bleeding. This often occurs because you are not ovulating despite making lots of estrogen. Estrogen acts like fertilizer on a lawn—it makes the uterine lining grow. Meanwhile, you are producing less progesterone due to lack of normal ovulation. According to Dr. Victoria Maclin, reproductive endocrinologist and assistant professor of obstetrics and gynecology at Rush Medical College in Chicago, "progesterone matures the lining. It holds the excess stimulation of estrogen in check, which allows the lining to slough off properly. Without the progesterone, unopposed estrogen will cause excessive and often very clotty bleeding."

Excessive bleeding or spotting intermittently can be a sign of an abnormality unrelated to menopause. The worst-case scenario is that the unusual or excessive bleeding indicates a malignancy in the reproductive organs. Most often, however, it is the sign of other, more benign conditions: fibroids, polyps, or nonmalignant tumors. On occasion, it may also be the result of a miscarriage or ectopic pregnancy.

"Fibroids are very common during perimenopause because estrogen stimulates their growth," adds Dr. Maclin. "Therefore, fibroids often get much larger during the initial stages, when estrogen levels in some women are unopposed. However, they tend to shrink on their own *after* menopause when estrogen levels have declined."

> "I had heavy bleeding because of fibroids. My doctor told me that if I managed to go through menopause without a hysterectomy, there was a good chance my fibroids would shrink. And they did. Just after my periods stopped, my uterus went from the size of a grapefruit down to the size of a walnut."

Hormones

Once other medical problems have been ruled out, there are a number of routes you can take to handle excessive bleeding. Taking progesterone in the second half of the cycle has helped reduce the bleeding for some women.

> "Sometimes I would bleed for ten to fifteen days, so my doctor said I should try progesterone pills. I'm going on my fourth month and I really like it. It's changed everything. I take it for ten days beginning on the sixteenth day after I start bleeding. I don't have any bloating at all until a day or

two before my period, which is perfectly acceptable. My period is four to five days long, with a little spotting at the end, but there is no prolonged agony, which is great."

Taking progesterone can be a tricky business, however. When it works, it's great, but it does not work for everyone.

"I went on progesterone for two months and it made me feel very uncomfortable, not like myself. I felt like I was working on two cylinders rather than six and I wasn't alert. I felt spacy so I finally went off it."

Other medical options for controlling heavy bleeding resulting from anovulatory cycles while providing reliable contraception at the same time include low-dose birth control pills, which reregulate the cycle and produce the reduced menstrual flow typical among birth control users, and the Progestasert IUD, which delivers topical microdoses of progesterone directly to the uterine lining and avoids the emotional and mental side effects common to oral synthetic progesterone.

Alternative Therapies

A number of women I talked with were helped quickly and effectively by acupuncture. It not only reduced their bleeding, it also regulated their cycle.

"My last period was one of the heavy ones, so I had an acupuncture treatment. The bleeding stopped immediately within an hour of the treatment."

Others were helped by homeopathy.

"I have fibroids. And my periods were just awful. My homeopath gave me two remedies and my periods stopped."

Gui Pi Tang, a Chinese herbal formula, slows heavy bleeding. So do shepherd's purse and blessed thistle, herbs that can be taken independently, either in the diluted homeopathic form or as a tincture, three days before your period. This is problematic, however, if your periods are irregular, because you won't know when to take it.

Invasive Procedures

A more invasive procedure to curtail bleeding is a D&C, or scraping of the uterine lining. Another is an ablation, in which a ball heated by electricity sears the uterine lining and destroys most of it. A third procedure is the laser burning of the uterine lining.

A hysterectomy, or removal of the uterus, should be the last resort. We simply do not know enough about all of the functions the uterus performs to remove it without a compelling reason. For example, for a lot of women, uterine contractions occur with orgasm and removing the uterus severely curtails sexual pleasure.

For decades, American physicians have readily recommended hysterectomies. Nearly one-third of American women will have their uterus removed before menopause, and half will have it removed within their lifetime. American statistics are significantly greater than those of Great Britain and other European countries. So beware. Make sure you know your options before you choose to go under the knife.

If you do decide to have a hysterectomy, you may want to preserve the cervix. Pressure on the cervix during intercourse is often an important source of sexual pleasure and can contribute to the experience of orgasm. The cervix also produces prostaglandins, which affect the nervous system in numerous ways. And certainly, should you require a hysterectomy, do not have your ovaries removed unless there is absolutely no alternative. Currently, about half of the women over forty who undergo a hysterectomy also have their ovaries removed. Many unenlightened surgeons think that since they are operating anyway, they might as well prevent any possibility of ovarian cancer. But the ovaries keep producing important hormones for most, if not all, of our lives and should not be removed preventatively, especially given that only just over 1 percent of women ever get ovarian cancer.

If you have been bleeding heavily, have your blood tested to make sure you are not iron-deficient. Sufficient iron is necessary for the blood to carry oxygen to the cells throughout the body. If you are deficient, the best food sources of iron include dried fruits, prune juice, beans, liver, rare red meats, green vegetables, nuts, peanut butter, whole-wheat breads, and cereals. Picolinate capsules and liquid iron preparations provide good supplementation while generally producing less constipation than iron tablet supplements.

Ultimately, bleeding ceases permanently. And while a woman may experience negative symptoms during The Pause, losing her periods is rarely one of them. According to a number of European studies, more than 70 percent of women are relieved when their periods end.

"I guess I just never accepted it as a lack of femininity or anything. I didn't feel like I was less of a woman. Actually, I love not having a period. It's so nice not to worry about whether you're going to get it on a vacation or not. Quite frankly, it's a relief."

This relief was expressed among women born in different generations and among different cultures. Studies of Central European, Turkish, Iranian, North African, and Arab women revealed that most of them welcomed the cessation of their periods.

The negative aura surrounding menopause has little to do with the end of monthly bleeding. Rather, it is the result of the accompanying physical and emotional discomforts and the outmoded but still prevalent view that women past childbearing age are of no use either to themselves or society.

Further Information

Janine O'Leary Cobb. *Understanding Menopause*. New York: Plume, 1993.

6

Mirror, Mirror on the Wall

Our culture celebrates youth and beauty as if women were perennial contestants in the Miss America Pageant. Products from cars to alcohol use sexy females to boost sales. My nine-year-old cousin recently visited me, and to keep her busy, I suggested she put on a mud facial mask—I thought she would have fun playing with the gloppy green mud. I was stunned by her eager response. "Yes, yes," she cried. "Anything for beauty."

We seem to know, at a very young age, whether we are pretty enough to join the "in crowd" or are too plain to be desirable. From early on, we compare ourselves with models in magazines, on television, and in the movies who often have eating disorders and large plastic surgeon bills. We delight in comments like "You look beautiful" and "What a great body you have."

Now, as we enter The Pause, our bodies are undeniably changing. No matter how many aerobic classes we take a week, gravity is having its way. For a lot of women, these changes are alarming.

> "I can't remember the last time a construction worker whistled at me. I miss it now that it's gone. It's funny, even if I didn't feel good that day, a whistle would make me feel better."

> "The hardest part of getting older is that when I walk into a room, nobody looks up anymore."

You may find yourself unconsciously feeling jealous of a teenage daughter. You may even be fighting with her more, not realizing that competitive feelings may be setting you off.

> "I was walking down the street with my daughter the other day and a couple of men stopped and looked. Suddenly I became aware that they were looking at *her* and not at me. It was a little hard on me. I felt proud of her, but at the same time, I felt bad about myself."

Because we have learned to value ourselves for our beauty, as our breasts begin to sag and wrinkles appear, many of us feel depressed, anxious, or worthless.

> "My body is never going to be what it was. It makes me mad that we've been brainwashed to think about our bodies in very unfortunate ways."

If we tie our sense of sexual vitality to youth and vigor, as our bodies begin changing we may fear the loss of our sexual selves, and some of us do lose our partner's interest at this time. Generally this occurs not because we've become unattractive, but because we reflect back to him his own aging process. To deny his aging and confirm his virility, many men seek out a younger woman. While it is probably not hormonally based, this is the male menopause we hear so much about.

For women who have based their lives on childbearing and child-rearing or on their physical attractiveness, menopause can be a most difficult time. With children gone and youthful beauty fading, a major life transition is catalyzed. If a woman can't expand her skills and sense of self, she may begin to feel lost and worthless. Women who are able to redefine themselves using their own standards, and not those society dictates, usually fare best.

"I figure, I have to make an adjustment. I'm not going to be as attractive anymore and I'm just going to have to get used to the idea. I have to be happy in myself. And I judge others differently, too. I sound like my mother. I want to connect with someone because he or she is a good person. Otherwise, my bullshit detector goes off and I have no need for them."

Possibly one of the least talked about issues is the loss of a kind of power that occurs with the loss of youthful sexual attractiveness. Without even realizing it, many of us have received prompt or extra attentiveness from male clerks or salesmen throughout our lives, or perhaps we were readily assisted if the car broke down or when trying to negotiate an armful of groceries, simply because we were young and physically appealing. I can remember a computer operator who, unasked, offered to analyze an entire research project I was working on during my senior year in college. I'm not sure I would have gotten the same response from him today. With age comes invisibility. This means that we may have to learn to do more things on our own, or reevaluate our priorities.

"I turned gray in my late thirties, so I lost that allure early on. But I've never minded. A certain respect came with that change, and quite honestly, I find being regarded with respect much more fulfilling than being seen as sexually alluring."

"Sure, nobody flirts with me when I sit next to them at a dinner party the way they used to, but I don't find it such a big loss. I have much more interesting conversations now, and I really enjoy that."

WEIGHT

There is no doubt that middle-age spread starts appearing just around the time of The Pause. One study from the Massachusetts Institute of Technology showed that two-thirds of women who were of normal weight before a natural menopause and 95 percent of the women who had been obese had gained weight. One of the most common complaints during The Pause concerns difficulty controlling weight. Women talk about how it is harder to take off weight and easier to put it on. Those who have battled weight problems for years, and those who haven't, agree that something is noticeably different.

"I've been about a hundred twenty pounds since I was seventeen years old. Now I'm close to a hundred thirty. Everything seems to have settled around the middle, so this is the first time in my life I'm doing sit-ups. But no matter what I do, the weight seems just to settle there. For the first time, I understand people who have weight problems. I always thought, 'It can't be that hard to lose weight. All you have to do is stay off fattening food and do a little exercise.' But it's not true."

"Weight has been a lifelong issue for me. It's been up and down. Three years ago I got down to my goal weight, but almost as soon as I got down there, I started piling it back on. Now I've put most of it back and I'm having difficulty staying even. It feels like I'm always fighting it, always gaining weight. In the past, after a diet, I'd plateau and stay in the same place. Now the weight comes back immediately."

"Around two years ago, when I was forty-six, my whole body started changing. I felt thicker in the waist. I'm working harder to keep ahead of weight gain, but the returns are diminishing. It's a real battle. Sometimes I can take off a few pounds, but the weight returns so rapidly."

Both men and women gain weight with age. But for women the issue is more sensitive. For example, in a July 1991 survey I did for *Longevity* magazine I found that while almost as many men as women had gained weight during their late thirties and early forties, only one-sixth of the men felt their weight gain had negatively affected their sexuality. Nearly half of the women did.

Men are drawn to a woman's beauty, but women are attracted to a man's power and status. While many men gain power with age, women often lose beauty as it is culturally defined. How frequently have you seen a gorgeous woman on the arm of a powerful but homely man? More often than you'd probably care to admit. How many times have you seen the reverse? Rarely. Given how much of our sense of self-worth comes from our physical appeal, it is no surprise that gaining weight can be incredibly traumatic for many women.

Both men and women gain weight because metabolic rates decline about 2 percent per decade throughout adult life. This accounts for much of the buildup of extra flab. But between the ages of forty-five and fifty-four, women gain significantly more than men. It appears that this weight gain can be directly tied to hormonal changes. Progesterone increases metabolic levels, and during The Pause our levels of progesterone are decreasing. But more importantly, a gain in weight may be nature's way of protecting us, as fat cells turn into miniature hormone factories, busily converting androgens to estrogen. Finally, the tables have turned, with health and feeling good on the side of the majority of women who are not ultra-thin.

While some extra weight is a real plus during The Pause and afterward, too much weight increases the risk of a heart attack and other medical problems. For example, women who are very overweight may make too much estrogen. Once they stop ovulating, they no longer produce progesterone. This means the estrogen is unopposed and they have a higher risk of developing cancer of the uterus.

Consequently, there is a difference between aging gracefully and giving up the battle. Rather than trying to recapture the figure you had at twenty-five, you may need to accept a new standard, a comfortable weight that doesn't have to be maintained by deprivation, but one that promotes good health.

"Although I'm thirty pounds heavier than my ideal weight, my self-esteem is not wrapped up in it the way it used to be. I'll cut my fat intake because I don't want to die of a heart attack, but as far as my weight goes, I'm not feeling bad about it."

Some women gain considerable weight as the result of going on hormones.

"I've gained about fifteen pounds since I went on hormones. And I do notice, as I get close to my period, I crave sweets and salt. Nothing is more delightful than Fritos and a Hershey bar."

"Premarin and Provera worked fine for me. All the symptoms and hot flashes went away. The low-level depression went away, but I put on about ten pounds—mostly fluid—and I wasn't thrilled about that."

According to Dr. Arpels, this need not happen. "Many women gain weight because they have been put on too high a dose of estrogen too quickly and the body holds on to fluid because it can't adapt. If their weight gain is not a part of the aging process, lowering the dose of estrogen and then gradually increasing it over time should solve the problem."

Sometimes, however, the rise in renin substrate in the liver that results from taking estrogen *orally* increases the uptake of salt into the cells and causes bloating. In this case the solution is to change the form of estrogen you are taking. Premarin has a greater effect on the liver, so another type of estrogen might be better. Using the patch or letting the Estrace tablet dissolve under your tongue has less effect on the liver because you are not absorbing the estrogen through the digestive tract. You should also cut down on your salt intake if you are retaining water.

For some women, it is the progestin that causes the bloating. "Progestins and progesterone can increase salt retention," says Dr. Arpels. "It is also a smooth muscle relaxant and may affect the intestines, causing abdominal bloating. If the progestin is the cause, you may have to decrease the dose. Also, some of the progestins have male hormonelike properties (Norlutate, Norethindrone) and produce a muscle bulking-up effect that can cause weight gain in some women. In this case you would want to change to a different progestin or to natural micronized progesterone."

According to a recent Australian study, hormone replacement therapy *prevented* an increase in *abdominal* fat. The fat instead seemed to be distributed more evenly around the body. Besides helping women feel less unattractive, this pattern of weight distribution is different from that which has been correlated with women who have heart attacks.

Exercise

The highest weight gains take place among women with the lowest exercise levels. Whereas dieting lowers metabolic rates, exercise increases them, which means you not only burn off calories while exercising, but you burn calories faster during the rest of the day as well. Exercise also works better than very-low-calorie diets, which may lack necessary nutrients.

For weight loss, aerobic exercise is best. Change your lifestyle so that you can work in a minimum of twenty minutes per day, or, one hour three times per week, of walking, jogging, dancing, or swimming. Your long-term vitality and health require it. Also, whenever possible, walk up steps rather than taking the elevator. Don't grab the closest parking space; look for one a few blocks away. Jog in place while watching television. It all adds up to being in better shape, inside and out.

Diet

While we also need to reduce our calories *somewhat* to make up for the lowered metabolism that occurs with aging, it is really eating the right foods and cutting out the wrong ones that is essential to maintaining weight. Most importantly, reduce your intake of fat. If you eliminate fried foods, butter, ice cream, whole milk and most cheeses, poultry skin, bacon, sausage, salad dressings, and nuts and cut down on salmon and red meats, you will notice a difference in your weight. Substitute nonfat milk (low-fat milk is still high in fat) and part-skim cheeses, poultry without skin, and meats with as little fat as possible. (Better yet, cut out all or most animal flesh. It's good for your heart, bones, and weight. But more about this in Chapter 10.)

If you do eat meat, choose the leaner cuts from the leg or loin. Drain the fat during and after baking, broiling, or roasting. Skim fats off before making gravies and sauces. Substitute lemon juice, chicken broth, wine, and vinegar for butter, margarine, and oils whenever possible. Use nonfat yogurt instead of mayonnaise or sour cream. Of course, you can cut back on fats further, but just these few changes will make a tremendous difference.

For basic energy needs, eat complex carbohydrates: rice, pasta, whole-grain breads and cereals, starchy vegetables, dried beans, and peas.

Don't cut out the fun things. If you have one large meal, let yourself enjoy it. Then balance it with a smaller one. Eat smaller meals in general—three large meals, if divided into six small ones, will produce less weight gain. Allow yourself two bites of that obscene dessert—the first and the last. Then wait a number of days before you indulge again. Drink lots of water. Water will keep you hydrated, feeling full, and encourages a positive fluid balance.

But mostly, we need to reevaluate our ideas of beauty, especially when they make us slaves to calorie-counters and put us in a constant state of vigilant sacrifice and deprivation. It's crazy to let your sense of self and your joy in life be dictated by movie casting directors and fashion magazine editors. If you eat for your insides rather than your outsides, you will feel happier and healthier—which means you will look more attractive.

"We need to be able to say, 'What can I do to make this body healthy and happy?' Loving it and accepting it for what it is, rather than trying to have it stop in some time warp."

"I've gained about fifteen pounds, but I dress well and I still get a lot of attention from men."

It's all about taking our bodies seriously. We cannot mistreat them any longer. Our bodies deserve to be given what they need: diet, exercise, and care. They will continue to serve us well if we take the time to treat them properly.

"You just can't ignore your body and go out and do anything you want to do. I realize I have to take care of my body if it's going to keep me going. My back has been bothering me so I bought a new desk chair and mattress. After seventeen years one deserves a new bed, don't you think? Now my body is demanding a very different kind of attention and I'm responding."

If you want to, you can use this time of change to catapult yourself to a higher standard of health and fitness. As a result of changing my diet and exercise regime, I now feel better and stronger than I have in years.

"I think if my menopause had been easier, I wouldn't have started exercising or have changed to a low-fat diet. I know I'm a lot healthier for it, but it *has* been hard work."

HAIR

Our hair responds to hormonal changes. For example, some women lose hair immediately after childbirth. Hair can also thin when The Pause begins. If your hair follicles are deprived of estrogen, your hair can get drier and start falling out. Baldness, however, is extremely rare. Lack of estrogen also can cause a loss of pubic hair.

While hair on the head and pubic area may thin, a woman may notice more, darker, or coarser hair growing on her chin, upper lip, abdomen, or chest. Most women who experience this increased hair growth notice it after their periods have stopped. According to Dr. Albert Kligman, professor of dermatology at the University of Pennsylvania School of Medicine, "By ten years or so after menopause, hirsutism on the chin and lip is extremely common, especially for women of Mediterranean origin who have dark skin. You don't see it because they shave it or pluck it or wax it or something. But it's very common."

For many women, this increase in facial hair begins *early* in The Pause.

> "One of the first things I noticed was these long coarse hairs growing on my chin. I had no idea what was happening and it worried me."

Androgens are the hormones responsible for the male's heavy body hair, as well as male baldness. While androgens are predominantly male hormones, all women have them as well, and they account for these patterns of both increased and decreased hair growth.

Estrogen and androgens counteract each other. As estrogen levels decrease and no longer oppose the androgens, the androgens have a greater effect on the body. Also, during the period of erratic hormonal production in The Pause, androgen levels may surge intermittently. The result can be losing hair on the head (especially for genetically predisposed women) and gaining it elsewhere.

In addition, about half of us have special cells in the tissue of our hair follicles that cause hair to grow when levels of LH (luteinizing hormone) are increased—and remember, LH levels rise as we go through The Pause. It appears that, once stimulated, these hair follicles need only small amounts of androgens to keep producing this heavy hair growth. Consequently, hair growth can continue at an increased level even after production of androgens has dropped.

If facial hair bothers you, bleaching as well as professional or self-administered electrolysis can hide or eliminate it. But choose your electrologist carefully. There is no schooling requirement for an electrologist, and one who is inadequately trained can cause scarring or ingrown hairs.

Once facial and body hair has started to thicken, taking estrogen will not reverse the process, but it can prevent the problem from developing further. Because progesterone is an antiandrogen and blocks androgen receptors, some women find that using a natural progesterone cream twice a day during the second half of the cycle, or daily after cycles stop, can decrease facial and body hair within six months.

Women who have lost hair may find that estrogen in combination with an antiandrogen in addition to applying Rogain (a hair growth stimulant) to the area, increases new hair growth. One study out of Washington, D.C., showed that this treatment combination produced significant new hair growth for 93 percent of the participants with the remaining 7 percent still experiencing some improvement.

Ho Shou Wu is a Chinese herb that can be used when hair has thinned.

SKIN

Acne often appears during adolescence, pregnancy, and menopause—all times of hormonal change. When the relative balance among estrogen, progesterone, and androgens is upset, you can get acne. The likely cause is a relatively elevated level of androgens. I never had acne as an adolescent, but when I was pregnant and now during The Pause, I am seeing in the mirror what I missed.

Because of its antiandrogenic effects, some women find that using a natural progesterone cream during the second half of their cycle controls their acne. Dr. Kligman suggests Retin-A to clear up acne resulting from this hormonal imbalance. "I work with a lot of women who have blackheads, whiteheads, or some inflammatory lesions that occur as the result of hormonal changes that precede menopause. It's usually nothing severe. I have them use Retin-A and it stops the acne cold. In the beginning, there may be some skin irritation when using Retin-A, and you have to keep out of the sun, but there are no other side effects."

Men and women experience skin changes with aging that have *nothing* to do with hormones. As we age, the supporting fibers under the skin start to break down. The layer of fat cells beneath the skin declines, and we tend to look drawn. Fair-skinned women notice dark spots or liver spots, particularly on the backs of their hands; dark-complexioned women notice white spots.

Dryness and loss of elasticity, however, *are* skin changes linked to reduced estrogen.

"My skin texture has changed. The changes seem more rapid at this point. I notice the lines in my face more. My skin seems to be thinning and it's much drier."

Some women also notice that they bruise more easily as their estrogen levels drop—but this can also be a sign of vitamin C deficiency.

While supplemental estrogen does not seem to be the

fountain of youth for the skin that it was purported to be when it first came on the market, it does tend to make the skin a little plumper and reduces excessive dryness both by increasing skin collagen and by holding moisture in the skin.

Despite estrogen, skin is going to age. And even though susceptibility to aging is partly genetic, there are some things you can do to keep your skin in its best condition. First, quit smoking; smoking is antiestrogenic, deprives skin of oxygen, and increases wrinkling. Second, keep out of the sun, and wear a hat or use sunscreen when you *have* to be in the sun. Next to smoking, the sun is the major aging agent for the skin. Third, drink at least four glasses of water a day to replenish the 60 percent of the body that is made of water. When I asked my seventy-four-year-old aunt how she kept such youthful skin, she told me her secret: water, water, water.

According to Dr. Michael Klaper, director of the Institute for Advancement of Nutrition Education and Research in Manhattan Beach, California, "If women are having dry skin, I strongly advise them to sharply reduce, or better yet, eliminate meat and cheese from their diets. These contain acids that can cause dry, flaky skin and even contribute to wrinkling and premature aging. Next, I have them add two teaspoons of flaxseed oil to their diet every day. You can find it in the refrigerated section of health-food stores. Don't cook with it, because it breaks down when heated. Use no more than two teaspoons daily on salad, vegetables, or bread. Within a week their skin gets a nice luster to it and their hair gets shinier."

Use a good water-based moisturizer on your face and oil your skin frequently, especially after bathing. Or add oil to your bath when you plan to soak awhile. One woman swore by the sesame oil she rubbed into her body before bedtime.

Of course, you always have the option of succumbing to cultural pressures and getting your face lifted. Plastic surgery is currently expanding more rapidly than any other medical subspecialty. However, if we resist the pressures of Madison Avenue and the media to have our faces lifted and our tummies tucked, we may be able to create a new image for women over fifty—one that is positive and life-affirming. This doesn't mean that we should stop trying to look attractive. It feels good to look good. But we can look good and still look our age.

> "I dress better in some ways than I did when I was younger. Not flashy, but I look more like me. I'm much more concerned with being distinctively me rather than being a caricature of an attractive woman. For example, I've let my hair grow long."

> "I've changed how I dress, how I present myself. I feel much more attractive than I have ever felt before. I used to think that to adorn oneself was shallow. Now I think of dressing myself as a way of looking at myself from the inside out. I never wore makeup, but now I do. I'm discovering how I want to look and I'm enjoying the process."

Luckily, our culture is beginning to change. We baby boomers, because of our sheer numbers, are making an impact. Lauren Hutton, who is near fifty, has more modeling work now than ever in her career. The Institute for Standards Research of the American Society for Testing and Materials (the Greenwich Mean Time of body shapes) is finally recognizing that women's bodies change, and is developing new size standards for women over fifty-five.

> "I like the idea of shedding those skins and valuing who I am on the inside rather than the way I look from the outside. Five years ago, I thought those wrinkles around my

eyes were me. Now I feel less and less that my skin is who I am and more and more that it has to do with what's inside of me. I feel I am growing and that's exciting. I used to be real reluctant to wear my glasses anywhere except driving because I thought I looked awful in glasses. Now I realize that I can see better with glasses and things look prettier. That's more important to me than what I look like. And I like myself for starting to think this way."

"I had an absolutely horrific menopause. But if you asked me if I could take a pill and do it all over again without a glitch, I'd say no. I think it has made me so much richer, more compassionate and real. My life was easy, superficial. I never talked about the real stuff of being human. Now I can get down and dirty. I can stand in the bedroom with nothing but my socks on, fanning myself. I look ridiculous, given that I'm the woman who used to take her socks off first before going to bed so I didn't look silly. Now I let myself be just the way I am and I love it. I think that if I had just taken a pill, I'd still be trying to look pretty, maybe even getting a face lift."

By the year 2000, one-third of American women will be over fifty. These numbers mean force, both economic and social. We will have the clout to create a new feminist movement, encouraging society to value us for our experience, wisdom, and mature beauty rather than for a youthful face and a body like a twenty-five-year-old's.

Further Information

Naomi Wolf. *The Beauty Myth*. New York: Doubleday, 1991.

CHAPTER

7

Life Between
the Sheets

What many women fear most when they think of menopause is an end to their sexual desirability and their sexual pleasure. As a result many of us may be afraid to let others know The Pause is upon us.

> "I have found myself reluctant to tell my married women friends that I've started going through menopause because I assume that they will tell their husbands and I don't want the men to know. I'm afraid they will stop seeing me as a sexual woman. I don't want to be seen as desexed; a grandma; perfectly safe and without any allure."

Since sexual attractiveness is so essential in defining a woman's self-worth in this culture, and since sexuality is so thoroughly intertwined with reproduction, it is easy to see why many of us fear that we will lose our sexual desirability once we can no longer bear children.

However, sexual desirability and sexual satisfaction have

little to do with the ability to get pregnant. Certainly sexual attraction is a biological force that is fundamental to continuing the species. But just because our work of bringing babies into the world has ended does not mean that the physical and emotional joys of sex have to terminate as well.

Nevertheless, because menopause signals the shutting down of our reproductive abilities, it *can* have an impact on sexual functioning. If we do not need to reproduce, we do not need to have intercourse, at least not from an evolutionary point of view. Consequently, sexual complaints are commonplace during The Pause and afterward.

The good news is that the difficulties we encounter will not reduce sexual satisfaction for about 80 percent of us. For the rest of us, there are safe and effective solutions.

ATTITUDINAL BARRIERS

For some women, the sexual changes experienced may not be due to hormones. Psychological factors play a strong role in sexuality and, for certain women, menopause can be the long-awaited excuse to abandon sexual activity.

"I'm experiencing very low desire. I mean, it's not like my libido was excessive before. Sex was never something I felt comfortable about and I had a tough time with my body and all that."

Wanting to stop having sex is common among women who rarely found sex pleasurable in the first place. This group includes women who were sexually abused in their youth, who were indoctrinated about the sinfulness of sex, or who are involved with an inconsiderate or unknowledgeable lover. In addition, relationship problems can create major obstacles to sexual desire, especially when anger has built up over the years. When you feel that you have no power anywhere else in the relationship, you may find that the only power you hold is to say "no" in the bedroom.

Women who have been married for many years may not feel they have the right to terminate sexual relations. A partner accustomed to an active sex life may balk, blame, and induce guilt. But a good sexual relationship should provide sexual pleasure for both partners. If you are dissatisfied, if the sexual relationship offers you no benefit, you will have no incentive to continue it merely for the pleasure of another. But there are things you can do about it, if you choose, as we will see later in the chapter.

Single women have unique problems when it comes to sexuality. Women will outnumber men by approximately four to one in our later years, so finding a male partner of one's own age is not exactly good betting odds for heterosexual women. Certainly younger men are available, and many women are abandoning their preconceived notions that an older, more mature man is the only suitable partner. Others are expanding the parameters of their sexuality by exploring lesbian relationships. Still, as we age, many of us will find ourselves uncoupled. Consequently, submerging our sexual desires or replacing the loving hand of a partner with our own may remain the available alternatives, especially given the increasing dangers of AIDS and other sexually transmitted diseases.

> "There is no time in my life for sex. And, quite honestly, I don't miss it. Given the hassle with AIDS and other diseases, sex just seems to be more trouble than it's worth."

Finally, some women were raised to believe that sex should end at a certain age, that older women who are sexual appear degraded or comical. They may be embarrassed about sexual feelings and quash them in favor of perceived societal expectations.

These and numerous other psychological reasons can make the termination of sexual activity desirable. For these women, menopause may finally offer the permission they need to reclaim their bodies and step out of the sexual arena.

Certain drugs such as barbiturates, antidepressants (like Prozac), phenothiazines, and diuretics can affect desire, lubrication, and sexual functioning. Chemotherapy and certain medical conditions decrease the level of sexual interest as well. And then there is the effect of changing hormones.

From a hormonal point of view, The Pause can directly affect sexual desire, lubrication, arousal, and orgasm. Let's take lubrication first.

LUBRICATION

Blood moves into the pelvic region and congestion causes secretions to seep through the semipermeable membrane of the vaginal walls. As estrogen levels decline, we see reduced blood flow to the vagina. The result is a change in lubrication. Besides a difference in the quality of lubrication, 40 to 60 percent of women experience an increase in the amount of time and stimulation required to become lubricated. And when they do become lubricated, the amount produced is far less than in their younger years. For some women, this change in lubrication is the first harbinger of The Pause.

"I have dry spells. Suddenly during intercourse, the lubrication just kind of cuts off. And it's like the Sahara Desert."

"The quality of my lubrication can vary considerably. Sometimes it can be kind of thin, while at other times it's the way it used to be."

Without sufficient lubrication, some women may doubt their level of sexual arousal.

"I didn't know this about myself, but I guess I sort of used the fact that I was lubricating as a confirmation that I was turned on. When my lubrication changed, it became a more intellectual experience. I started to think, 'Gee, if I'm not lubricating, I must not be turned on,' which wasn't the truth. But I started to feel insecure and that definitely impacted our sexual relationship."

Be aware that antihistamines and some decongestants do not discriminate. They dry out all the mucous membranes, including those of the vagina, so avoid them if you are experiencing vaginal dryness.

PAINFUL INTERCOURSE

Not having enough lubrication, or lubrication that is insufficiently viscous, can make intercourse painful.

I remember that in the very early stages of The Pause, before I knew what was happening, my vagina would remain dry regardless of what we did or how much time we took. For a while, I found myself avoiding sex. It was just too uncomfortable. Then David and I started to use Astroglide, a lubricant available in most pharmacies that is specifically designed for sexual use. That made a big difference. But after a couple of years, intercourse was painful or it burned no matter how much lubrication we used. I didn't know it then, but the vagina is rich with estrogen receptors. When deprived of estrogen, the lining gets thinner and over time, with continued deprivation, loses elasticity. Thinner vaginal tissues means less cushion against the friction of the thrusting penis. The result can be a mild burning sensation during lovemaking and sometimes for hours or even days afterward. You may also feel a greater need to urinate after sex.

"I'm having really painful intercourse. No matter how much lubricant I use, it's still not comfortable."

"It wasn't burning or terrible, it was just more like a pain that I wasn't used to feeling."

This pain or burning with intercourse can begin long before your gynecologist is able to detect any changes in your vaginal tissues. Many women question their caring for their partner or look for other psychological causes when sex becomes painful and their physician can find no physical basis for it.

Why the change in estrogen creates pain with intercourse for some women, but not for others, is unknown. But if this is your experience, it does not mean you have to stop having sex. It does mean that you will probably have to make some adjustments if sex is to continue to be enjoyable.

Lubricants

You may have to extend foreplay, skip intercourse, or use a considerable amount of additional lubricant. Good water-soluble lubricants include Astroglide, K-Y jelly, and Calendula (marigold) cream, gel, or ointment. And while sex therapists have been advocating water-based lubricants for years, because oil-based products are not secreted from the vagina as easily and can cause vaginal infections, some women don't find water-based lubricants viscous enough to protect them. They prefer Vaseline, coconut oil, or the oil from vitamin E capsules. (But please remember, you cannot use *petroleum-based* products with latex condoms. They weaken the latex.)

> "I've tried a number of things, but I like Neutrogena sesame oil the best. It's not sticky and doesn't dry up quickly."

Women who prefer not to use a lubricant with intercourse recommend using Replens, a suppository you insert in the vagina every other day to keep the tissues moist. A small research study showed that the regular use of Replens made a significant improvement in vaginal dryness and comfort during intercourse. Other women advocated rubbing the oil from vitamin E softgels or inserting vitamin E suppositories in the vagina once a day to twice a month, depending on need. It's important to experiment until you find the product that works best for you.

Zinc has a positive effect on lubrication and vaginal secretions. The recommended daily allowance is 15 milligrams per day. Nuts, seafood, meats, wheat germ, and oats are all rich in zinc.

Hormones

While a lubricant will solve discomfort due to lack of lubrication, it won't reduce pain caused by thinned vaginal tissue and decreased elasticity. Estrogen, however, addresses these problems. Estrogen keeps the vaginal lining plump, lubricated, and pain free. If the only problem you're experiencing during The Pause is discomfort while having sexual intercourse, you could insert estrogen cream directly into the vagina a few times a week. Although some women notice a difference after their first application, others may have to use the estrogen cream for a month before they respond. One study from Denmark showed that one-quarter of 1mg Estrace tablet inserted vaginally twice a week also gave relief from sexual discomfort.

In sufficiently low doses, Estrace cream inserted vaginally can even be used safely by women who have had an estrogen-dependent cancer. "Every woman is different, so we give women very low doses of estradiol cream vaginally, and then check the estradiol levels in their blood," reports Dr. Lila Nachtigall, director of the Women's Wellness Division, Department of Obstetrics and Gynecology, at New York University. "If the estradiol in their blood doesn't go up, then they may be able to use it safely even if they have had an estrogen-dependent cancer. We are also using a new product, a vaginal ring, experimentally. It emits only five micrograms of estradiol daily, much less than a woman could apply herself. If it works, it would be approved for all women and blood tests wouldn't be required."

A 1- or 2-percent testosterone cream that can be made up specially by a pharmacist, or natural progesterone cream, can have the same effect on the vaginal tissues as estrogen cream. The only drawback to these creams is that they can be messy.

"Intercourse was painful. But I was impatient and didn't stay on the estrogen pills long enough. Then I tried Estrace cream every other night. It was a bit messy and a definite deterrent to sex on *those* nights—but hey, it wasn't like I was having sex on a daily basis anyway."

Hormone creams were not designed to be lubricants. They are not only ineffective as lubricants, but the man's urethral opening can absorb the cream and, while probably not harmful, we do not know how this *small* amount of hormone may affect him.

Herbs

The herb chasteberry can revitalize the vaginal tissue and diminish pain with intercourse, but it generally takes a few months to experience positive results.

"I went through menopause about three years ago and I was having more and more pain with intercourse. My gynecologist said she could actually see the changes on a slide taken of some vaginal cells. She had me make a tea out of chasteberry. After about six months of drinking it a few times a day, the pain just wasn't there anymore."

Phytoestrogens, plant estrogens found in certain foods, appear to help restore the health of vaginal wall cells. Women who supplemented their daily diet with 45 grams of soya flour or 25 grams of linseed, foods high in phytoestrogens, showed a significant improvement in their vaginal tissues after six weeks of supplementation. The positive effects were sustained as long as the diet was maintained.

SEXUAL TOUCH AND SENSITIVITY

Some women respond to The Pause with changes in skin sensitivity, which can affect sexuality. They may find that they like a harder stroking or a gentler touch than in the past. Areas that used to be aroused when touched may now not respond or may actually feel irritated. This is particularly true of the breasts, which frequently become far more painful both at midcycle and during the last week before menstruation begins. To decrease breast pain, take 400 to 800 international units of vitamin E each day. You might want to take a lower dose during most of the month and then raise it during the point in your menstrual cycle when your breasts are most tender.

During The Pause, some women find the clitoris uncomfortably sensitive, or don't find stroking it as arousing as it once was.

"I'm orgasmic mostly from penetration, but I've also enjoyed clitoral stimulation of all different forms. Now, though, I don't enjoy it as much as I used to. It doesn't feel the same."

"My clitoris feels less sensitive and the stimulation is certainly not as intense."

"I used to enjoy receiving oral sex. Now it's okay, but it's not anything that I really enjoy and I haven't been orgasmic with oral sex for a while."

Some women notice lessened sensation upon deep thrusting. With decreased estrogen, the pressure sensors in the cervix may become less responsive. Some women experience this as a great loss in sexual pleasure. However, estrogen supplementation will increase their responsiveness. In fact, estrogen appears to have a positive impact on all aspects of sexual functioning during and after The Pause.

ORGASM

With decreased hormones many women find that their orgasmic response changes. Changes in orgasm can be the result of reduced estrogen, which limits pelvic blood flow, or the result of insufficient testosterone. While some women find that their orgasms get more intense over the years, more common changes include taking longer to reach orgasm, reaching orgasm less frequently, or having less intense orgasms.

> "I've experienced a change in the physical experience. It takes longer to reach orgasm and my orgasm is less intense. Now I'm waiting for my memory to fade so I don't notice."

For most women, however, these changes in orgasm are not significant and do not necessarily diminish sexual enjoyment. In fact, while women may experience less intense orgasms, they often describe them as gentler and sexier.

> "My orgasms seem to last longer. So while there may be a drop in intensity, there's an increase in duration. I used to always have more than one orgasm when we made love and that has changed, too; it's harder to get there the second time. But there is a softness to my orgasms that is really wonderful. It's very different from the frenetic, intense orgasms of yore, but they're really quite lovely."

Occasionally, women experience painful contractions with orgasm, almost like a muscle spasm. "A lack of estrogen can cause painful contractions during orgasm," according to Dr. William Masters of the Masters and Johnson Clinic in St. Louis. "These contractions are quite real and there is nothing psychological about them. But if you take estrogen in some form, you can eliminate them."

CONTRACEPTION

We all know about menopausal babies. And while few women get pregnant during The Pause, it certainly remains a possibility.

"At forty-one, I made a conscious decision to have a child because I'd waited so long. It all happened so fast. In December I started getting hot flashes so I decided that if I was going to get pregnant I had better do it right away. In January, I was pregnant."

If you want to ensure that you *don't* get pregnant, you should continue to use contraception until one year after your last period. If you are not in a monogamous relationship, you need to use condoms even after that. AIDS and other sexually communicated diseases know no age limits. Until you have been with a partner in a monogamous relationship for six months and have tested negative on the AIDS blood test, you should avoid anal sex and use latex condoms with a spermicide containing nonoxynol-9.

If you are experiencing pain with intercourse, condoms may increase your discomfort. Condoms may also interfere with a man's erection as he grows older and his responses become more fragile. However, women are the fastest-growing subgroup contracting AIDS and are more vulnerable than men to all sexually transmitted diseases. If condoms are problematic, stick to manual stimulation unless you are certain your partner is disease-free. Unprotected sex is like Russian roulette. The odds may be in your favor—but if you lose, the consequences can be grave.

POSTMENOPAUSE

While symptoms like hot flashes, fatigue, and sleep disturbances tend to diminish in intensity and then finally disappear within a year or two after the last menstrual cycle, if a woman is not manufacturing sufficient estrogen in her fat cells, changes occurring in her sexual organs will keep progressing unless she does something to remedy it.

Without sufficient estrogen during the postmenopausal years, the vagina becomes less elastic and shrinks. This means that during arousal, the most interior end of the vagina no longer balloons out as far as it did in the past. The vaginal lining will change to an almost paper-thin consistency. The result is that unless the vagina is kept stretched, intercourse will be painful if you should stop having intercourse for an extended period and then try to start again. This can be ameliorated, however, within about six weeks if an estrogen cream or hormone replacement therapy is used in addition to stretching the vaginal walls with a dilator or dildo.

To stretch the vaginal walls, begin with something narrow, like a Q-Tip or your pinky. Lie on your back with your knees raised; lubricate the vagina and the object to be inserted, then bear down—as if trying to push something out of the vagina—as you slowly insert the object. This bearing down actually relaxes the vaginal opening and makes insertion easier. Leave the object in for fifteen minutes. Then push the object in and out of the vagina to help stretch the anterior wall. Once this is comfortable, use objects of increasing width and length. Dildos come in many different sizes and can be purchased by mail if no legitimate sex stores are located in your area. Carrots, zucchini, and cucumbers can all be rounded down to the desirable size. Just peel them or wash carefully to remove any insecticides—or place a

condom over them—and let them warm up to room
temperature before inserting. There is also a theory that
hormones in the male ejaculate can help protect the vaginal lining, and that having sexual intercourse at least
once weekly may help prevent or ease painful intercourse.

Masturbation

If you do not have a partner or are not sexually active
with your partner, it is in the best interest of your vagina,
and possibly your psyche, to continue masturbating. So, after so many of us have been brought up to feel guilty and
abnormal if we *did* masturbate, a New Jersey study now
shows that regular masturbation after menopause keeps
the vagina healthy. Masturbation helps maintain the lubrication process, and masturbating with something inside the
vagina like a dildo or cucumber keeps the vaginal walls
stretched.

In addition, many women need the physical release
masturbation affords. It makes them feel better about
themselves. They feel less tense. And while masturbation
cannot replace a loving partner, it can provide its own
kind of sexual pleasure. Consequently, it is often enjoyed in
addition to partner sex.

Miscellaneous Changes

Reduced estrogen affects the reproductive system in
other ways. After menopause the sex flush on the neck and
chest that had occurred with orgasm often disappears. Because of the loss of subcutaneous fat—fat under the skin—
the breasts and nipples become smaller and flatter over
time and the outer lips of the vagina lose their plumpness.

The reduction in protective padding may result in sensitivity or soreness of the clitoris in certain intercourse positions. Estrogen will counter all of these sexual changes, and for many women the sex flush will return.

SEXUAL DESIRE

Many women fear that menopause means loss of sexual desire, as well as sexual desirability. And the truth is that at least 35 percent of women *will* experience a reduction in sexual desire during The Pause or afterward. In recent research, Dr. Norma McCoy, a psychologist specializing in hormones and sexuality at San Francisco State University, found, "The biggest decline in sexual intercourse took place during the one- to two-year period *before* a woman's last menstrual cycle. In addition, over fifty percent of the sixteen women we studied showed a decrease in sexual thoughts and fantasies during the years around menopause."

The loss of sexual desire can be gradual or sudden. Sometimes it occurs early in the process of The Pause, sometimes not until five or more years after the last menstrual cycle. For some women the effect is transient; for others, permanent.

"I used to have this burning desire to masturbate and also these very sexual thoughts about other women. Then suddenly, it all went away."

"I miss that intense feeling of sexuality, like if I don't have you right now, I'm going to die. It still happens every now and then, but generally only after we're already making love. It used to be that if Joe would walk around nude in our bedroom, I would kind of jump him. Now I still get great pleasure out of looking at his body, but I just don't have that same energy."

When we lack sexual interest, the immediate tendency is to assume the cause is boredom or relationship problems—and certainly most long-term relationships have their share of both. However, the genesis is likely to be psychological only when sexual and relationship problems have been long-standing. In those cases, marital or sexual counseling become the solutions of choice. Otherwise, a loss of desire on the woman's part is most frequently due to decreased hormones. According to Dr. Gloria Bachmann, associate professor of Obstetrics and Gynecology at Robert Wood Johnson Medical School in New Jersey, "Most sexual problems in this older population stem from ovarian hormone decline rather than interpersonal, psychological, or cultural problems."

Desire often abates when insomnia, hot flashes, and other symptoms of The Pause interfere with our energy and sense of well-being.

"I can't help it. When I'm nervous and irritable, I'm just not interested in sex."

Not feeling well is a major sexual inhibitor. So is pain. Women who are experiencing pain with intercourse caused by lack of lubrication or a thinning of the vaginal lining may find themselves avoiding sex. Sexual desire is likely to return, however, once the discomforts of the transition have passed or some form of treatment (estrogen, homeopathy, acupuncture, herbs, or lubricants) has stopped the symptoms. A study at Yale University, for example, showed that 90 percent of the women who had experienced a lack of desire before the study reported an increase in desire and sexual activity after being treated with estrogen for three to six months. If you are sleeping better, having fewer hot flashes, and feeling better in general, you are likely to be more interested in sex.

For more than a year I was so fatigued and drained of energy that sex rarely crossed my mind. Finally I went to a homeopath and was given the remedy Sepia, in the form of tiny pills. Within a few weeks, my old energy level and interest in sex returned.

"Since I've started on estrogen, my hot flashes have stopped. I sleep through the night. I'm not so tired and I find my sexual interest has increased."

"I'm taking the herb chasteberry and I've recently started acupuncture. Slowly I've been getting my sexual drive back, particularly around my former high times—at ovulation or just before my period."

A lack of testosterone, particularly bioavailable testosterone, can also reduce sexual desire. Our ovaries and adrenal glands each produce approximately half our testosterone supply. "We don't know why, but for approximately fifty percent of women, testosterone stops being produced in the ovaries at about the time of menopause," reports Dr. Barbara Sherwin. "The rest maintain normal ovarian production for some period of time." According to research conducted at the University of Massachusetts Medical School, most of this drop in testosterone occurs *prior* to the actual menopause, which is why many women may experience a lack of desire at this time. Women who have undergone chemotherapy, or who have had their ovaries removed, may experience a precipitous drop in testosterone—as well as sexual desire—virtually overnight.

There is no absolute level of testosterone necessary to feel sexual desire—as with estrogen, every woman has a different set-point. But if testosterone falls below your individual base level, you are apt to experience a decline or absence of sexual desire, a decrease in clitoral sensation, and an increased difficulty in attaining orgasm either through masturbation or with a partner.

According to Dr. Helen Singer Kaplan, director of the Human Sexuality Program at Payne Whitney Institute in New York, "No psychiatrist, psychologist, or internist can look at a woman who has *totally* lost her libido at the menopause and tell me whether this is organic or psychogenic because the clinical picture is identical. The sex centers are as easily shut down by depression as they are by a lack of testosterone. The only way to tell is to take loosely bound and free serum testosterone levels, which are easy to do. Any lab can do it. The results will tell you whether the woman needs psychotherapy or testosterone supplementation. However, some women may benefit from both."

Progesterone competes with testosterone for receptor sites. This means that even if a woman has sufficient testosterone, if she has too much progesterone, she may experience a lack of desire because the progesterone is filling up the receptors. These women may experience a lack of desire in the second half of the cycle.

"Some research shows that Premarin, the most popular estrogen pill, can decrease levels of bioavailable testosterone in some women," says Dr. Norma McCoy. "If you are feeling a lack of desire and are on Premarin, you might want to switch to Estrace or the patch."

If you are taking estrogen and your symptoms are gone, but you still feel a lack of desire, you may need additional testosterone. The safety of prescribing testosterone, however, is currently a controversial subject. There is fairly strong agreement that, in high doses, testosterone can produce facial hair, a lowered voice, weight gain, and acne, and can adversely affect blood lipid levels and the liver. The question is, how potentially negative are *small* doses of testosterone?

Dr. John Arpels says, "I generally prescribe a two-milligram tablet of testosterone two to seven times a week when appropriate. As long as the dose is below seventy-five milligrams per month, five percent or less of my patients experience any weight gain, hair growth, or acne."

Of greater concern is the effect of oral testosterone on cholesterol levels. One product on the market, Estratest, combines estrogen and testosterone in one tablet. Dr. Morris Notelowitz, president and director of the Women's Medical and Diagnostic Center and Climacteric Clinic in Gainesville, Florida, has been studying Estratest. "We compared the effects of Estratest and Estratab, which both contain esterified estrogen, but Estratest also includes testosterone. We found that the women on the combination treatment showed greater improvement on symptoms like depression, anxiety, and libido when compared to women taking Estratab, who also showed improvement, but not to the same extent. Secondly, the patients on combination treatment showed greater improvement in their bone density when compared with Estratab by itself. The only negative thing about the Estratest is that it *did* decrease HDL cholesterol (good cholesterol), although it remained within normative range. On the other hand, the Estratest significantly decreased triglycerides, which in some women is a particular problem. So the bottom line is you have to tailor your treatment to the individual, and Estratest has an important role in treating menopausal women, but not all menopausal women."

The effects of oral testosterone on masculinization or cholesterol are only one part of the issue according to Dr. Norma McCoy. "The real issue concerns the negative effects of synthetic hormones on liver proteins. We simply don't know enough about the long-term adverse effects of low doses of these synthetic hormones when taken orally. In addition, synthetic testosterone, like Premarin when taken orally, increases the liver's production of binding proteins which then selectively bind testosterone. When the testosterone is bound, it is not bioavailable, and it can't enhance sexual interest or anything else."

Testosterone can also be taken non-orally. Research shows that these non-oral routes have no negative impact on the liver or blood lipid levels. Upjohn used to make a sublingual testosterone, and though they no longer manufacture it, it can still be found in many pharmacies. A 1- or 2-percent testosterone cream can be made up by a pharmacist and rubbed on the inner labia every few days. And Depo-Testadiol or Depo-Testosterone can be given by injection. "I like to use injectable testosterone," reports Dr. Edward Lichten, "because it bypasses the liver and has less of an effect on blood lipid levels. I use it with women who are perimenopausal or postmenopausal, and with women who've had a natural or surgical menopause. Women generally receive an injection every four to six weeks, but some women take it as frequently as every three weeks or as infrequently as every three months depending on how fast they metabolize it."

"I started testosterone because I had my ovaries removed. My libido dropped dramatically, and since I enjoyed sex a lot, I really didn't like it. So I am getting injections of Depo-Testadiol every six weeks. I used to take pills, but I feel better on the injections. My husband gives them to me in the hip. Before I started the testosterone, I would feel sexual only after I was being kissed and touched and all that, but I never masturbated or felt interested in sex on my own. Now I anticipate it. I look forward to it and I initiate sex more like I used to."

Testosterone pellets that act for six months can be inserted under the skin, but this method is generally only used with women whose ovaries have been surgically removed. According to Dr. Victoria Maclin, one of the few physicians using testosterone pellets in this country, "Testosterone pellets don't improve cholesterol levels, but they don't make them worse. The women I have treated complain of either a diminished libido or a total lack of sexual desire. They also feel more lethargic and have less zest for life. Adding testosterone to their hormonal replacement, if their testosterone levels are low, restores their libido and improves their sense of well-being. And those changes have not been accompanied by increased hair growth, weight gain, or acne."

"Alza in California is creating a testosterone patch for men," offers Dr. Helen Singer Kaplan. "A woman would only need one-tenth of it, and it would be perfect for breast cancer survivors because it uses dihydrotestosterone, a compound which cannot be tranformed by the body into estrogen."

Regardless of the form in which you take testosterone, if you take it, you must be carefully monitored by your physician.

Not all women, however, are concerned about reactivating their level of sexual interest. Some women could not care less. With a declining sexual need, they find their energy turning in other directions.

"At about age fifty-eight or fifty-nine I started to experience a lack of desire. At first I thought it was an issue, but now I've decided it isn't. I still feel sexually excited every now and then, but I guess because there are so many other good things in my life, it's not that significant."

"First of all, my sexual energy has decreased a great deal. I used to feel I could have sex all the time. It was always on my mind and there was a sense of urgency. I no longer experience that very often. The kind of fantasy stuff we used to be interested in no longer does it for me. It's been a real shift and I've had to adjust to that. The funny thing is, I'm

not really missing it. It's not a big problem. We have begun
to move into the companionship part of our lives."

INCREASED DESIRE

According to a Danish study, 9 percent of women report
an *increase* in their level of sexual desire at some point during or after The Pause. A variety of factors can account for
such an increase. With no more fears of pregnancy, menopause can open whole new areas of sexual freedom for
some women. A new partner can revitalize a woman's
sense of her own sexuality, while for women in long-term
relationships, no longer having the children at home can
mean a second honeymoon.

"The office closes at five o'clock, and we have a glass of
wine and go for a walk on the beach. Then we come home
and make love, and afterward we have dinner. When our
son came home from college over Christmas, we really felt
deprived of that romantic time."

There are also hormonal reasons for increased desire
during The Pause. Dr. Norma McCoy examined sexuality
across the life span and made some interesting discoveries.
"We found a peak in sexual interest in women in their
early forties. Kinsey and his colleagues observed the same
thing, but he ascribed it to the culture, believing that it
took that long for women to overcome the sexual inhibi-
tions instilled in youth. But it appears that hormonal
changes may be the more likely reason."

Just as you turn up the volume when you can't hear the
television, when estrogen levels decrease, the body tries to
stimulate more estrogen by turning up the FSH and LH.
In addition to stimulating the production of estrogen, the

increased LH and FSH stimulate special cells in ovarian stromal tissue to make testosterone. Some women are more efficient than others at producing testosterone this way. It may be that these women are the ones most likely to experience this increase in sexual desire.

Sometimes increased testosterone production occurs erratically, just as during puberty when you suddenly get acne and feel incredibly horny.

> "In the last two years, beginning when I was forty-six, I've become very sexually interested. I listen to my friends talk about how they're disinterested and I know that my estrogen level is declining; but if anything, I'm having an increased desire for sex."

If you should be in the lucky minority—with both a loving partner and an increased level of desire—enjoy your good fortune. You can never tell how long sound health and a positive relationship will bring you such pleasures.

MALE PARTNER PROBLEMS

The primary reason that sex stops for women in heterosexual relationships may have nothing to do with menopause. It may be determined by the woman's male partner. One study found that men showed less sexual interest in their late forties and fifties than women. And in another study, 80 percent of the women and 71 percent of the men believed the man was the one responsible for ending their sexual relationship.

> "I just last week said to my husband, 'I notice my sexual energy is down.' He answered, 'Yours is down? If you think yours is bad, you should see mine. Mine is the problem.'"

There are a number of possible reasons for this decline in male sexual interest. With age, a man requires more direct stimulation of the penis to get erect and it takes more time to attain an erection. Fantasy or just looking at his partner does not do it the way it used to. And a man is likely to have more difficulty maintaining an erection once he attains one. Thoughts or outside noises often intrude in ways they never did before. He also may not have an orgasm every times he makes love. All these changes are a natural part of a man's aging process, which can begin as early as in his forties or early fifties, or not until his sixties or later. But if a man experiences changes without realizing that they are normal, he may begin to question his love for his partner. He may blame his slower response on the fact that *she* is aging, that *she* has gained a few pounds, that *she* is going through menopause. And she may accept the blame, feeling that a change in the way she looks or feels, a change in her femininity, is somehow at the root of the problem. He may then look to a younger woman to rekindle the excitement and response he fears he is losing.

Sometimes the woman's menopausal symptoms do directly influence the man's more fragile responses. He may worry about hurting his partner if she has been experiencing pain with intercourse. Or he may grow more anxious and insecure about his own ability as a lover when she responds less quickly and lubricates less copiously. This insecurity may then affect his own sexual performance.

Regardless of the cause, many men simply choose to end their sexual relationship rather than confront the problems. For these men, it is easier to deny the subject and avoid the painful feelings and fears of losing their masculinity, which unfortunately, for many, is defined by the performance of the penis.

Most women abdicate to their partner responsibility for their sexual relationship. Men tend to be the sexual initiators. Women frequently feel more embarrassed or awkward when it comes to bringing the subject up. They worry about appearing critical or hurting their partner's ego if his erections or interest are problematic. However, if a woman does nothing and the man is in denial, the result is often a silent ending to sex.

> "I think it started with the fibroids. When they were quite large, sex was painful. He became fearful that he was going to hurt me. That about coincided with his prostate getting larger and some difficulty he was having with erections. We don't talk about it. He has chosen not to deal with the issue. In other words, we still don't have sex."

Once we understand that sexual response slows down with age, that both men and women need more stimulation to become aroused and to reach orgasm, that not having an orgasm every time may be commonplace, and that lack of an erection or pain with intercourse need not mark the end to lovemaking—we can relax, and adapt sex to fit our responses. Interestingly, when we are more relaxed, we tend to be more responsive.

Touching, cuddling, holding, and stroking become as important a part of lovemaking as orgasm—even more so over the years. This means that rather than putting sex in the deep freeze, we may have to change our expectations and behaviors.

> "There were times when we would make love and there would be no penetration. My husband would try, and I'd just tell him to forget it. Often he would masturbate me and then see if it was possible to come inside. If it wasn't, I would do a hand job or stimulate him orally, or whatever."

If intercourse becomes less reliable or less satisfying, manual and oral stimulation can take on greater importance. One study of sexually active males and females over age sixty showed that while 97 percent said they still enjoyed sex, only 9 percent said that intercourse was the most important part. Even when an experience does not end in orgasm, which will happen on occasion, and with greater frequency as we get older, sex can still be rewarding and thoroughly satisfying.

For more enjoyable sex, you may have to slow down and allow more time for lovemaking. Occasionally, to keep interest piqued, you might try to get out of the routine and make love during the afternoon or somewhere other than in the bedroom. Take a bath or shower together before making love. Rent an X-rated video or read some erotica either alone or to each other. Wear sexy lingerie to spice up the visuals. Perfume also enhances lovemaking for some couples.

If sex is a priority, show it by setting time aside for your sexual relationship. Squeezing in sex late at night after a full day when you are tired and have to get up early the next morning is not conducive to the best lovemaking. Make dates. Get dressed up and do things together. Go away for romantic weekends.

> "Sex is better when we go away for the weekend. With my hot flashes and the stress at work, we need to get away to relax and to really spend some time connecting together. Then the sexual part seems to come back."

Time to be intimate and time for sex are two very crucial factors in maintaining a lifelong satisfying sexual relationship. Keep the romance alive with small gifts, loving notes, or telephone calls. When you fell in love, you were probably lavishing attention on your partner. Putting energy back into your relationship will help to recapture those feelings. Set aside time to connect emotionally so that you *feel* like making love. Even twenty minutes a day of face-to-face talking, away from the TV or the children, can make a major difference in how close you feel to each other.

Some women find that even if they are not very desirous of sex, once they start making love they will get turned on. So when your partner initiates sex, rather than analyzing your responses, you might want to simply relax and see what happens.

"Although my desire level is down, when we make love, I have no problems with arousal. I tell myself, 'Just go ahead and make love and if you don't get really turned on, that's fine, but probably you will.' And I usually do."

It appears that during The Pause, sex is good both for your relationship and for your health. Dr. Winnifred Cutler, cofounder of the Women's Wellness Program at the Hospital of the University of Pennsylvania, observed that women who had intercourse regularly, once a week or more, had twice as much estrogen circulating in their blood as women who were either not sexually active or only active sporadically. Women with this more active sex life showed fewer negative changes in their vaginal mucosa and tended to have less severe hot flashes.

A study in Denmark showed that if women had sexual intercourse more than twice weekly at forty-five years of age, only 18 percent were likely to notice a decrease in sexual desire after menopause. In contrast, 47 percent who had had intercourse less than weekly noticed a decrease. These findings could be interpreted as "use it or lose it," or they may merely indicate that the higher the level of hormones you have circulating in your body, the more sexual you are likely to be. Either way, if sex is important to you, there are options available to treat interfering symptoms or depressed desire. And if you put a high priority on masturbation or sex with your partner, you can expect to maintain an active sex life for a long, long time.

Further Information

Lonnie Barbach, Ph.D. *Sex After 50* videotape. Institute for Health and Aging (800-866-1000), 1991.

———. *Erotic Interludes: Tales Told by Women.* New York: HarperCollins, 1987.

———. *Pleasures: Women Write Erotica.* New York: HarperCollins, 1985.

Good Vibrations—sells books and sexual products for women and couples. 1210 Valencia St., San Francisco CA (415-974-8990).

Bernie Zilbergeld, Ph.D. *The New Male Sexuality: The Truth about Men, Sex, and Pleasure.* New York: Bantam Books, 1992.

Bernie Zilbergeld, Ph.D., and Lonnie Barbach, Ph.D. *An Ounce of Prevention: How to Talk with a Partner about Smart Sex.* Audio tape. Fay Institute (800-669-0156), 1988.

8

Hormones:
Pros, Cons, and
New Options

Possibly the greatest source of confusion and concern for women going through The Pause is whether or not they should take hormones. We read newspaper headlines that fuel our fears, hear about estrogen causing breast cancer and other terrible things. Then we read about the incredible benefits, that it will save us from hot flashes, mood swings, heart attacks, and hip fractures. Some physicians recommend that every postmenopausal woman have hormone replacement; others say don't begin taking hormones until one year after your last period even if you are miserable, suffering from hourly hot flashes and insomnia.

Clearly, the information is confusing. If symptoms are compromising your physical or emotional well-being, or if you are at serious risk for getting osteoporosis or cardiovascular disease, hormones can be very effective. But how do you decide what is right for you?

"Hormone replacement seems like an incredible snake pit. Because of my kidney transplant I'm on drugs to suppress my immune system, so I am more prone to cancer. On the other hand, since I take Prednisone, I'm more prone to osteoporosis. So I think I should take hormones for the osteoporosis, but on the other hand I don't want to take them because of the cancer, so I'm stuck."

Each of us needs to find a personal solution to our unique set of circumstances. What works for one woman may not be at all appropriate for the next. For example, with some guidance, the woman quoted above got a bone scan to see whether she was losing bone mass. Her scan came out normal. She decided to get a scan every year; if she wasn't losing bone density, she had no reason to go on hormones. With information, she had found a rational way out of her dilemma.

NO HORMONES

In the past, women were not permitted to take estrogen if they'd had an estrogen-dependent cancer, blood clots not caused by an injury, liver disease, gallbladder disease, diabetes, or hypertension, or if they smoked.

The thinking, however, has changed. Replacement hormones are considered particularly beneficial if you smoke. They do not affect diabetes. As long as you don't take them orally, you don't have to worry about gallbladder disease. If you have had blood clotting problems, you can take hormones, provided your clotting factors are normal. Except for the synthetic estrogens found in birth control pills and possibly Premarin, women with hypertension are now candidates for estrogen supplementation or replacement, since estrogen generally helps lower high blood pressure by relaxing the muscle walls of blood vessels. And even women with past histories of estrogen-dependent cancers are being treated for sexual discomfort with very low doses of Estrace cream.

HORMONE REPLACEMENT THERAPY

Hormone replacement therapy (HRT) refers to estrogen and progesterone taken in combination. This can be done in a couple of different ways, as we will discuss later. HRT was designed for the *postmenopausal* woman, the woman who has stopped cycling and has her uterus intact. Originally, estrogen was given alone and the result was a devastatingly high increase in cases of cancer of the endometrium, the lining of the uterus. This happened because estrogen was continuously building up the uterine lining, but without the progesterone, this lining was never sloughed off as naturally occurs every month during our reproductive years.

While HRT consisting of estrogen and progesterone is appropriate for the postmenopausal woman with a uterus, many of us are having our worst symptoms while we are still cycling. At this time we are producing estrogen and progesterone on our own. Since HRT creates a regular, but *artificial* cycle, our own erratic hormone production is likely to cause midcycle or breakthrough bleeding. Breakthrough bleeding is an annoyance, but more than that, it can be a cause for medical concern—a possible sign of uterine cancer, cervical cancer, or other serious problems. When you bleed midcycle, your physician should do a uterine biopsy or vaginal ultrasound (if your uterine lining is four millimeters or less in thickness) to ensure that you are only bleeding in reaction to the hormones and that there are no abnormal cells. These procedures can be time-consuming, expensive, and unsettling.

Women who want to take hormones but who are still cycling have a few ways of getting around this dilemma: low-dose birth control pills, estrogen supplementation, or progesterone supplementation depending on the particular hormonal imbalance.

LOW-DOSE BIRTH CONTROL PILLS

Low-dose birth control pills override your normal cycle. They act on the pituitary gland in such a way that you no longer produce any estrogen or progesterone of your own. The birth control pills supply all of your hormones. The FDA has recently deemed low-dose birth control pills safe for women until the age of fifty who haven't had gallbladder disease, hypertension, or blood clotting problems and who don't smoke. Birth control pills have the added advantage of controlling excessive bleeding and also virtually guarantee that you won't get pregnant.

> "I was on birth control pills in my twenties and I had no problems with them, so when my gynecologist suggested them as a solution to my hot flashes and emotional symptoms, I jumped at the idea. And I'd have to say, I've had no problems since I've been on them."

While some women do well on birth control pills, others do not. It may be difficult to find a pill with the right estrogen-progesterone balance for you. The wrong balance can mean terrible PMS symptoms or menstrual cramps.

> "I took the lowest-dose birth control pill possible for two weeks and I felt horrid. I was depressed, nauseated, tired, and bloated. And I put on weight."

Another drawback is that low-dose birth control pills contain synthetic estrogen, and the synthetic estrogen used is 70 to 100 times stronger than the "natural" estrogen used in hormone replacement. This means slightly increased chances of developing hypertension (high blood pressure) and of having a stroke. Low-dose birth control pills can also have a negative impact on sexual desire for a lot of women.

ESTROGEN SUPPLEMENTATION

Estrogen supplementation refers to taking additional estrogen to supplement the amount you are producing on your own. You simply keep track of your symptoms to determine when in the menstrual cycle you experience them, and then start taking the estrogen a day or two before the symptoms would normally kick in. This way you are raising the level of estrogen so that it stays above the set-point.

For example, initially you might need only half a dose of estrogen every other day for the last two weeks of the cycle. As symptoms change, you might benefit from a higher daily dose during the second half of the cycle, or you might find a small dose in the first half of the cycle also necessary. However, since your own hormone levels may surge at times, it is helpful to know the symptoms of too much estrogen so that you can cut back on the supplementation when appropriate. Too much estrogen can cause weight gain, water retention, tender breasts, headaches, and nausea.

This whole idea of taking estrogen without progesterone is quite new. The increase in uterine cancer that occurred when estrogen was used alone left the medical community reeling. Prescribing estrogen alone became taboo. However, while you are still cycling on your own, you are producing sufficient progesterone and do not have to add progesterone to your regimen until your periods are more than two months apart. However, supplemental estrogen is not appropriate for all women who are cycling regularly. According to Dr. Mark Glasser, head of OBGYN at Kaiser Permanente in Northern California, "If you are having heavy bleeding, you probably are not producing enough progesterone and therefore are not a candidate for taking estrogen alone."

Estrogen supplementation has been a godsend for women in high-powered positions with responsibilities that require them to operate at peak performance mentally, physically, and emotionally. With estrogen supplementation, relief from symptoms is generally rapid—from a couple of days to within six weeks. I have recently started taking a quarter tablet of Estrace sublingually a few days before I ovulate and a quarter tablet twice a day during the ten days before my period. At this point in The Pause, I find it more effective than other approaches for handling the mental fog and the irritability, which have worsened over time.

"I feel much better since I went on estrogen. In fact, I don't know what I would do if I had to give it up."

"I was under tremendous stress. My mother was dying, my son was having terrible problems at school and I was having hot flashes umpteen times a day. Everything felt like it was upside down. I was at that breaking point where I just couldn't do it naturally. So I took hormones for a few months. All my symptoms went away and I felt wonderful."

Regulating estrogen supplementation can be tricky and often requires small adjustments in dosage over time as your own hormone production changes. It means working with a knowledgeable, dedicated physician who is willing to devote the considerable time necessary to fine-tune your hormonal regimen. Without the proper guidance and expertise, you may join the ranks of those who are not able to adapt to hormones.

"I started bleeding irregularly at thirty-five. For years I had all sorts of symptoms but no one put it together until I started having horrific hot flashes at forty-five. First I tried a normal dose of Premarin and Provera, but that didn't do anything. For two years I tried different hormones: Estratest, the estrogen patch, but nothing that worked for anyone else worked for me. Finally I found a physician who had me insert the estrogen tablets in my vagina and now, for the first time in four years, I'm virtually symptom-free."

FORMS OF ESTROGEN

Let's explore the variety of ways you can take estrogen. Most commonly, estrogen is taken orally, in pill form. Estrace and Ogen are prescription pills which are structurally exactly like your natural estrogens. This means they have the same chemical structure as estrogens made by the ovary. Women seem to have fewer problems with these pills than with conjugated equine estrogens such as Premarin, which while also natural because it is made from the urine of pregnant mares, contains some estrogens only found in horses. Since 10 to 15 percent of Premarin does not have the same molecular structure as human estrogen, it cannot be used by human estrogen receptors, and the normal (.625-milligram) dose may not be as effective as the equivalent dose of Ogen or Estrace. The benefit of Premarin is that it comes in a greater variety of dosages, and most of the research done on estrogen has been done using Premarin because it was the first estrogen available forty years ago.

Oral estrogen presents problems for those women who do not absorb estrogen very effectively through the digestive tract. Even when they double or triple the estrogen dose, many of these women still experience symptoms of low estrogen. They may do better if they take the estrogen non-orally.

There are a few simple non-oral routes for supplementing estrogen. Estrogen can be taken transdermally, meaning through the skin. It can also be absorbed through the vaginal walls, or dissolved under the tongue, leaving virtually no aftertaste. All of these methods avoid some of the negative effects that can occur when the hormone hits the liver directly from the digestive tract. If it enters via the bloodstream, the initial impact on the liver is less intense. This means reduced risk of clotting problems and of increasing hypertension in susceptible individuals.

The Patch

The patch is a recent development in estrogen replacement. It consists of a small round pouch a couple of inches in diameter that adheres to the skin of your stomach, thigh, or buttock like a Band-Aid. The estrogen in the patch is absorbed through the skin. You change the patch approximately twice a week. Otherwise, you keep it on when you shower, bathe, or swim.

> "I started on the lowest-dose pill but I continued to have the hot flashes, so my doctor raised the dosage. And then he raised it again and my breasts became so tender that it hurt to walk. Finally he put me on the patch, which I'm still on. I have to say, for me it's the most satisfactory."

In addition to easing the impact on the liver, the patch, unlike pills, dispenses estrogen continuously throughout the day and night. This more closely mimics natural estrogen production and can be important for women who are particularly sensitive to getting a burst of hormone just after they ingest the pill.

The patch, however, has drawbacks. The first is that it currently comes in only two sizes.

"The patch was terrible. I felt like a helium balloon—getting more and more bloated."

"There are creative ways to get around this limitation," claims Dr. John Arpels. "You adhere the sticky side of a Band-Aid to the middle of the back of the patch. This occludes part of the backing, which reduces the total surface area available for absorbing the gel contained inside. A new patch, which can be cut into various dose-appropriate sizes, will be available in three to four years."

The patch is also considerably more expensive than oral hormones. But the biggest drawback is skin reactions. "There are two reasons for skin sensitivity to the patch," claims Dr. Arpels. "One is that alcohol from the gel inside the patch pocket often accumulates on the backing of the patch during storage. This alcohol can cause a skin rash. If you air the patch for five minutes before applying it, the excess alcohol evaporates and doesn't bother the skin. The second is that the patch is such a good adhesive that it keeps oxygen away from the skin. Irritation can occur because the skin is not getting enough oxygen. So if airing the patch doesn't resolve the problem, then move the patch every twenty-four hours to a different site on your buttocks, where the skin is thickest."

Estrogen in a gel form (Estrogel) is popular in France. The woman squeezes a tube and measures the gel out on a special ruler, varying the dosage to fit her needs. Then she rubs it into her skin. Unfortunately, it is not yet available in the United States, but it should be soon.

Vaginal Absorption

The vaginal walls are excellent for absorbing estrogen, and taking the estrogen this way also avoids that first large dose that hits the liver when taken orally. Estrogen in cream form can be inserted vaginally, but has the drawback of being messy and a deterrent to sex on the nights used, unless inserted after lovemaking. Estrace tablets that are usually taken orally can be inserted in the vagina. Taking estrogen this way seems to have all the positive effects of the patch. Moreover, it is so effective women need only about a quarter of the oral dose.

"I had to take three milligrams of Estrace daily to control my hot flashes and rage. Now I can get the same effects with only one milligram when I take it vaginally instead of orally."

However, some women find vaginally inserting tablets messy and annoying. A little will leak out of the vagina and onto your underwear. Also, because it is best to insert the tablet before bed so that less will leak out, it can be an inhibitor to nighttime lovemaking unless it is the very last thing you do before you fall asleep. If this is a problem, dissolving the tablet under your tongue will generally provide the same positive effects.

PROGESTERONE

Once you stop ovulating or your periods occur less than every second month, if you have a uterus, you must take progesterone along with the estrogen.

Progesterone protects the uterus. Women taking a combination of estrogen and progesterone have the same or lower rate of endometrial cancer when compared with women *not* taking hormone replacement. In many cases when there is a hyperplasia, an overgrowth of abnormal cells in the uterine lining which can be a precurser to cancer, a few months of progesterone may remedy the problem, and the woman will not need to get a hysterectomy.

Progesterone can be given alone to those women who have a relatively higher level of estrogen production due to poor or no ovulation. The progesterone is generally taken for twelve days during the second half of the menstrual cycle to mitigate nausea, dizziness, and extremely heavy menstrual flow.

A natural progesterone cream can also be used to oppose relatively high estrogen levels in the last two weeks of the menstrual cycle. You rub the cream into a hairless area of the skin, where it is best absorbed. However, the cream is difficult to measure out in any reliable way, and should not be used to counter estrogen as a replacement hormone after cycling has stopped.

"Heavy bleeding has been my main problem, but since I started taking progesterone my periods have become much lighter."

Once natural periods cease, the progesterone can be discontinued or estrogen can be added to the regimen.

Some physicians are now recommending progesterone even for women who have had a hysterectomy because they believe the breasts need progesterone on a cyclic basis as well. Some doctors even believe that women who are not taking estrogen should take an injection of progesterone or a twelve- to fourteen-day cycle of pills at least once a year, in order to oppose the estrogen that may be naturally manufactured in their fat and other cells—either that or they should get a periodic uterine ultrasound or biopsy.

Progesterone comes in a few synthetic forms called progestins. The most commonly prescribed are Provera, a synthetic version of progesterone, and Norlutate, a progestin resembling testosterone. Progestins are structurally different from the progesterone we naturally produce. As a result, many women experience negative side effects. The major reason women stop taking HRT is because of these negative reactions. You may be reacting to the progestin if you feel fatigued, are retaining water, have overly tender breasts that feel full, experience increased vaginal dryness, or have a lessened libido.

> "The last week of my cycle, when I start taking the progesterone, I know that my breasts are going to hurt. My breasts are so sensitive that I cannot stand to have my nipples touched. And Bev loves to touch my nipples, so it's really uncomfortable to make love during those times."

But the most pervasive and problematic complaint women have about the progestin is that it causes their moods to range from enormously irritable to deeply depressed.

> "I felt suicidal on the progesterone. Everything looked black. Then twenty-four hours after I stopped it, I felt like a new person. I knew it was the drug because nothing else in my life had changed."

> "Even though the Provera stopped my heavy bleeding, I felt anxious and frightened and I had these horrible weird

dreams. When I walked into my doctor's office and she asked how I was, I burst out crying, so she took me off it immediately."

"I get these mood swings when I take the Provera. I feel cranky and headachy and start to feel real sorry for myself."

Remember, when you take the progestin, receptors are taken over by the higher levels of progesterone and are not free to use the estrogen. The brain, deprived of the estrogen, produces PMS-type emotional symptoms. However, if you take a little extra estrogen on the days when you are also taking the progestin, you can mitigate the symptoms. Also, taking or increasing your intake of vitamin B-6 to between 100 and 300 milligrams per day during the days when you are taking the progestin can sometimes stem the negative side effects.

TWO HRT REGIMENS

Generally, estrogen is taken every day. In the past, estrogen was prescribed only three weeks out of the month, which cut down on the incidence of endometrial cancer because the total amount of estrogen being consumed was reduced by one quarter. When progestin is added, estrogen can be taken every day, which has been a boon to women who experienced symptoms on the days they were off the estrogen.

The progestin is generally added to the estrogen in a manner that mimics the cycle of a woman during her reproductive years. What this means is that after taking the estrogen for fourteen days, you start the progestin. (Since you are no longer having periods on your own, you can begin the progestin on the first of every month, for simplicity's sake.) For the next ten to twelve days, you take the estrogen and progestin together. Then you stop the progestin but continue the estrogen. A few days after you stop the progestin you are likely to have a period, but the bleeding will probably be light and generally will diminish or stop as the years go by.

Because this hormonal bleeding feels disconcerting or just plain annoying to many women who have stopped menstruating, and because so many women have adverse reactions to the progestin, a second form of hormone replacement therapy has become available. In a form similar to birth control pills, a little progestin is added to the estrogen on a daily basis. Less is known about this regimen, but it apparently protects the uterus as well as the method that imitates the natural hormonal cycle. The major difference is that menstrual bleeding is less likely to occur or is considerably lighter. One-third of women taking the combined dose never have a period, and most of those who do, stop bleeding within three to six months. Only 20 percent have periods thereafter. If a woman has fibroids that are bothersome, this combined HRT method also seems to have a less negative effect. Fibroid growth under this treatment regime is unusual. In addition, some of the negative mood reactions are reduced because of the lower daily dose of the progestin.

"Finally after a year of intensely awful hot flashes, I cried uncle. I never take pills, not even aspirin, but I decided to take little doses of estrogen and progesterone every day with no breaks. I have normal periods and it's wonderful. I still have some premenstrual symptoms, but I actually feel like a free woman because I almost never get a hot flash."

This combined dose of HRT, however, has some problems. Women who are recently menopausal have a higher likelihood of experiencing breakthrough bleeding with this method. Some women get headaches from the progestin, even when taken in small daily doses. Also, there is some concern that the breasts require the progestin on a cyclic basis and that this continuous dose may not ultimately be as good for them. Finally, there is mounting evidence that after a few years on this combination method, breakthrough bleeding occurs more frequently, requiring women to face a new round of uterine biopsies. As a result, the combination method is not recommended until a woman is at least three years beyond her last natural menstrual period.

NEW FORMS OF PROGESTERONE

Because of the side effects of oral progestins, alternative approaches to obtaining the necessary progesterone to protect the uterus are being explored.

Progestasert is an IUD that is authorized for contraceptive use, but it may also be ideal for the postmenopausal woman because it delivers progesterone directly to the uterus. Unlike oral progestins, the progesterone in the Progestasert is identical to that produced by the woman's body. Dr. Roger Lobo, professor of gynecology at the University of Southern California, has carried out some research on the use of Progestasert for women in mid-life. "In pilot studies using Progestasert with menopausal women," says Dr. Lobo, "we found that sufficient progesterone to protect the lining of the uterus was delivered, but the small amount registered no measurable changes in the blood. This means there were no systemic effects and hence none of the common side effects women can get from the progestin."

The major drawback to the Progestasert is that it has to

be replaced yearly, and since it is a rather large IUD, this can be a painful procedure. But there are ways around this difficulty. "We reduce the discomfort of inserting the IUD," says nurse practitioner Patricia Baldwin, codirector of a women's health care practice in Palo Alto, California, where over 5,000 Progestaserts have been inserted, "by first applying topical benzocaine gel to the cervix, which makes it less sensitive to an injection of a local anesthetic. The local anesthetic numbs the cervix and significantly reduces the pain of inserting the IUD." Also, if ahead of time you take Motrin, or another antiprogestiglandin to relax the uterine muscle, this can help reduce cramping while the uterus is accommodating to the IUD.

Due to bacterial contamination that can increase a woman's chance of developing pelvic inflammatory disease, the Progestasert should only be used by women in stable, mutually monogamous sexual relationships.

Natural micronized progesterone pills, synthesized from a soybean extract, and less frequently derived from the wild Mexican yam, seems to cause fewer emotional side effects than the synthetic progestins. "Micronized" means that the hormone is treated so that it will not be destroyed during the digestive process.

Natural progesterone is a fairly new product, but research indicates that when 200 to 300 milligrams of natural micronized progesterone is taken orally, ten to twelve days a month, not only is the uterus protected, but there is no negative effect on cholesterol levels. It is also less apt to cause the depression, bloating, breast tenderness, and loss of libido that are common with the synthetic progestins. In fact, a rise in libido is often reported. A Parisian study of natural progesterones showed appreciably positive effects on depression, anxiety, and hot flashes. Natural progesterone also helps to prevent sugar cravings in susceptible women.

Natural micronized progesterone is quickly metabolized, so it should be taken twice a day. Since it can also cause drowsiness in some women when taken orally, 100 milligrams should be taken with breakfast or lunch (absorption is increased when taken with food) and the remaining 100 or 200 milligrams at bedtime.

However, drowsiness can be reduced by taking the progesterone non-orally. According to Dr. Kathryn Morris, a physician in Northern California who specializes in hormone balancing for women, "When taken orally, natural progesterone is converted in the small intestine in such a way that it may cause drowsiness. When small doses are taken vaginally or sublingually, the digestive system is bypassed and drowsiness does not occur."

Natural progesterone can also be made into suppositories to be inserted vaginally. Dr. Roger Lobo has been studying natural progesterone taken by vaginal suppository. He reports, "The absorption is very good when natural progesterone is used vaginally. You get a very high local concentration in the uterus, higher than that achieved with the same dose taken orally, so it opposes the estrogen and protects the uterus. At the same time, it has virtually no systemic effects."

Unfortunately, natural micronized progesterone can be considerably more expensive than progestins, so you need to check the prices at the various pharmacies that prepare it. (Pharmacies are listed at the end of the chapter.) Also, dose regulation is not always as dependable as with the progestins, and most doctors are not familiar enough with them to feel comfortable prescribing them. But if you are being helped by estrogen, only to find the progestin a problem, natural progesterone may provide the answer you are looking for.

TAILORING HRT

The trick to effective hormone replacement therapy is finding a physician who can tailor treatment to your unique biochemistry. For example, some brands of hormones are more effective than others for specific symptoms or for certain women. At a particular level of estrogen, one woman may continue to experience hot flashes even though her vaginal discomfort has disappeared. Another woman might have the opposite reaction. Some women adapt to HRT within a few months and the side effects disappear. Others go from one treatment program to another:

"After a year of hot flashes every twenty minutes, no sleep, and feeling like I was going psychotic, I finally decided to try estrogen, but it didn't work for me. It handled the hot flashes and I got some sleep, but I was on the combination dose and after a few weeks I started to bleed. It felt really crazy to suddenly be menstruating again. And it didn't stop. I just kept dripping all the time. So they gave me a larger dose that I took every day and stopped for the last week. This time I felt really weird, like I wasn't inside my body, but living about six inches away from myself. And then I started to bleed again. So I tried the patch and I was allergic to it. Finally, I said forget it. I'll do this cold turkey for a while."

A physician who can adapt hormones to the individual is like a creative chef. Anyone can follow a recipe, but it takes someone knowledgeable and experienced who can add a little sugar when the tomato sauce is too acidic or who can ascertain just the right touch of garlic.

Treating menopausal women with a little of this or a little of that is still very unorthodox, but it makes sense given our unique individual biochemical makeups. A number of women I talked to were helped by this approach when more traditional regimens failed. The woman quoted above was ultimately aided this way:

> "I used Premarin cream for a while, and my vagina felt better, but I was worried that the estrogen was being unopposed. So now I take estrogen and Provera for five days a week and nothing for two. I have no bleeding and my vagina feels terrific. And I'm not afraid all the time about getting uterine cancer. I don't feel like I'm out of my body. I only have hot flashes occasionally. And it took just two or three weeks to kick in."

Some women do better if they take half the usual dose of estrogen every day or take it every second or third day.

> "I took half an estrogen pill for three days and developed the most horrendous set of side effects. The best way to describe it was a heavy-duty anxiety attack. My heart was pounding. My chest felt like it was in a vise. I felt really lightheaded, weak, and extremely anxious. So I dropped it to half a pill every third day and I felt much better."

"During times of stress or when a woman is taking an antibiotic or when she has a fever or diarrhea, she may need to increase the dose of estrogen for a few days," suggests Dr. John Arpels. "These conditions all utilize estrogen more rapidly. Also, if a woman is getting negative symptoms from the progesterone, she can increase the estrogen by 25 to 50 percent during the days when she is taking the progesterone to help tide her over. Some research in Europe is showing that you don't have to take progesterone every month to prevent endometrial cancer; every second or third month may work equally well."

In some cases it is possible to take no progesterone at all, but then it is prudent to get a uterine biopsy every year or two while on the estrogen. If a woman starts showing a hyperplasia, which takes years to develop into cancer, it can be treated very effectively, in most cases, with 3 months of continuous progestin. Of course, the woman probably stopped taking the progestin in the first place because of its negative side effects, so these three months of treatment, while relatively short, are likely to be uncomfortable.

If you are having difficulty adjusting to hormone replacement therapy, it would be a good idea first to drop the progestin or progesterone while you experiment to find the right form and dose of estrogen. Since uterine cancer is very slow in developing, there is no risk in taking the estrogen alone for a few months. Once you are comfortable on the estrogen, you can then experiment with different forms of progesterone until you have determined a good fit. With this approach you are dealing with only one variable at a time and can more clearly isolate any problems and address them specifically.

FINDING THE RIGHT PHYSICIAN

Now that you are armed with all of these treatment options, what happens when your gynecologist tells you that you are wrong: that you cannot take estrogen without progesterone even though you are still cycling; that you must take off one week per month from estrogen to avoid increasing the risk of developing endometrial cancer; that natural micronized progesterone is not a valid approach? What happens if your physician wants you to take Premarin and Provera because they are the most frequently prescribed hormones and you want to take Estrace tablets vaginally and natural micronized progesterone because this combination is likely to have the fewest negative side effects? What happens if you are having bad menstrual cramps, depression, or other adverse reactions to the traditional treatment approach, but you still want to take hormones?

When your physician is loath to try something new or venture into an area in which he or she is really not sufficiently experienced, do you cave in? Let's face it, you are not the expert on hormones—your physician is, or at least is supposed to be. It's easy to abdicate power when on unsure footing, and it can be difficult to counter a physician's self-assurance. But remember, your body is at stake. You are the one living day-to-day with The Pause or attempting to adapt to hormones that are not quite right for you.

You do have choices. If you and your physician have a long-term relationship and he or she is respectful of your views, you could suggest that he or she read this chapter and the reference books at the end, which have been included precisely for this purpose.

> "I brought all the information I had gotten at a menopause seminar to my doctor. He was thrilled to get it. It turns out that I am the only person at Kaiser getting testosterone and he had to special-order it for me, so at first it was a big deal. But now it's fine."

If providing your physician with information doesn't work, you could get a second opinion—not from just another gynecologist, but from a specialist in menopause. After all, you would not think twice about going to a cancer specialist if you had a skin malignancy, even if it was on your outer labia. If you had fibroids and your gynecologist recommended a hysterectomy, you might consult a second physician known to take a less invasive approach to curing the problem.

Don't let yourself be intimidated. Contact the North

American Menopause Society for the name of a menopause specialist near you (see "Further Information" at the
end of this chapter). Knowledge is changing so rapidly that
most gynecologists and family doctors can't keep up with
recent discoveries and theories about how to treat women
during The Pause. This is where the expertise of a specialist can make all the difference. Consequently, the physician
who may have been wonderful at delivering your babies
may not be your best choice at this point in your life. So
please, listen to your intuition. Don't let loyalty to your
physician get in the way of good care.

> "I really waited too long to get the proper care. I had been
> literally hemorrhaging every month for well over a year and
> I was constantly exhausted. But I was wary about changing
> doctors. I liked the fact that my doctor was a woman and
> she had become a kind of friend. I guess that was the hard-
> est part. I felt like a traitor, so I waited way too long before
> I was willing to go elsewhere to get the help I needed."

I had a patient who began to get depressed within a few
months of starting on hormone replacement therapy.
Nothing in her life circumstances could account for the depression. I thought the progestin she was taking might be
causing the problem. Being submerged in this research, I
agreed to call my patient's gynecologist to try to determine
an alternative treatment regimen. When I called, I suggested natural progesterone. I was informed that there was
no research data on it. I countered that there was. I was
told that I was wrong. I referred my patient to another
gynecologist who specialized in menopause.

Some battles are simply not worth fighting. The object
is to get the best health care possible, not to educate those
who believe they have nothing to learn. Your physician
should be your ally. If your doctor is not supporting you

adequately, you deserve the services of someone who can. After all, you are paying handsomely for it—in time, money, and reduced quality of life.

On the other hand, you need to be realistic. Because of the multifaceted role hormones play in almost every bodily function and the tremendous individual variability of hormone production, especially at this time in life, treating symptoms of The Pause is a difficult, time-consuming business. You may finally get it right only to go back into disequilibrium in six months as your own hormone levels again change. Consequently, you need to be patient, keep a daily diary of symptoms, and work carefully with your physician.

BREAST CANCER

Fear of breast cancer is a major deterrent to taking estrogen. If nothing else, the statistic that one out of eight women (13 percent) will get breast cancer is terrifying. I had avoided taking hormones because of this fear. However, it appears that this statistic has been grossly misrepresented. The truth is, according to a 1992 National Cancer Institute release on cancer statistics, that one out of eight women will get breast cancer in their lifetime if they live beyond age ninety-five, and the risk of developing breast cancer rises significantly with age. Up to age fifty, there is only a 2 percent risk of getting breast cancer. If you have not gotten breast cancer by age fifty, you have a 5 percent chance of developing it by age seventy. If you haven't gotten it by age seventy, you have a 4 percent chance of developing it by age eighty-five. Each year you are free of the disease, you leave the risk for that year behind. So now maybe we can all sleep a little better at night.

The next question is, exactly how much of an effect does taking estrogen have on breast cancer? The research studies on estrogen and breast cancer show contradictory findings. The divergent results are due to a number of factors. First of all, there are probably four different kinds of breast cancers, and estrogen may affect each type differently. Second, we really don't understand how estrogen is metabolized in the breast. Breast fat has the ability to make its own local estrogen independent of whether hormone replacement is given, and it may be this specific local metabolism that is related to breast cancer. Finally, different forms and doses of estrogen have been lumped together in many studies which may have confounded interpretation of the data. When all the studies are taken together, one analyst found a small heightened risk for developing breast cancer when estrogen is taken alone, but no increased risk when progestins are added.

According to Dr. Patricia T. Kelly, director of medical genetics and cancer risk counseling at Salick Health Care, Inc., and author of *Understanding Breast Cancer,* "Nobody has really been able to draw a straight line between estrogen and breast cancer. If estrogen were the culprit, why, in women not taking hormones, would we see a continued increase *after* menopause, when much of their estrogen production has shut down? Also, if we're dealing with a causative agent, we would expect the risk to go *up* with increases in dose for women taking the hormone. But it doesn't. We would expect it to go *up* the longer the woman is on hormones. Well, we have good data on women taking hormones for up to twenty years and the risk is not significantly increased. The risk also doesn't go *down* once a woman *stops* taking replacement hormones. I've researched this thoroughly and was amazed to find nothing more than an occasional study here and there showing a slight increase in risk."

While few experts believe that estrogen actually *causes* cancer, there is fair agreement that it may act as a fertilizer, meaning that if the beginnings of the weed are already in the garden, the estrogen may accelerate its growth.

"I took hormone replacement therapy for a year and then I developed breast cancer. Fortunately, it was microscopic, something they found on a mammogram. I had a lumpectomy and radiation treatment and I also stopped taking the estrogen because they found the tumor was estrogen-positive."

Looking at the data carefully, it does appear that there are a few factors that *increase* a woman's likelihood of developing breast cancer. An early menarche or a late menopause, after age fifty-five, are established risk factors for developing breast cancer. So is a first full-term pregnancy after age thirty. But other possible causes are confusing. Women with benign breast disease have been considered at risk for developing breast cancer, but, according to Dr. Kelly, "Only about three to five percent of women with benign breast disease, those who have what is called atypia, are at increased risk. Most studies have not distinguished between women with and without atypia, but have lumped them together. It's as if a drop of red liquid (atypia) were added to a glass of water (other types of breast disease), turning the water pink and making it look as if all women with benign breast disease were at increased risk. In the same way, most studies find that as a group, women who have had no children are at increased risk of breast cancer. However, at least one study shows that the increase in risk may be confined to those who are infertile due to progesterone deficiencies."

Breast cancer risk is probably a combination of individual hereditary predisposition and environment. 85 to 90 percent of women diagnosed with breast cancer have *no* close relative with the disease. But a history of cancer on *either* side of a woman's family, particularly having a mother or sister who had breast cancer before menopause, can increase the risk to 20 or 30 percent depending on how many close relatives have malignancies in one or both breasts.

But according to Dr. Kelly's research, studies today do not show that risk is *further* increased by taking hormones. "All I can tell you is that some studies find a *decreased* risk to women taking replacement hormones who have a mother or a sister with breast cancer, compared to women with similar family histories who are not taking hormones. And *most* find no increase in risk whatsoever. There is also no increased risk of developing breast cancer for women with benign breast disease when they take replacement hormones."

In addition, research shows that women who are taking estrogen when their breast cancer is diagnosed appear to survive the cancer better than those who were not taking estrogen. "We don't know if it's because women are getting the benefit of better observation from their physician," suggests Dr. Roland Young, associate professor of OBGYN at Baylor College of Medicine in Houston, Texas, "or maybe it's because these women are more concerned about the risk of breast cancer, so they are more conscientious about self-examining their breasts. But I believe it's possible that estrogen actually protects the breast. Some studies show that there is less progress to cancer when women who have precancerous lesions or benign breast disease take estrogen."

I must say that doing this research has quieted my concerns about estrogen and breast cancer. The studies that do show an increased risk in breast cancer for women on hormones demonstrate a very small increase. According to Dr. Graham Colditz, associate professor of medicine at Harvard Medical School, "Approximately one additional woman in one thousand per year will get breast cancer while on estrogen compared to women who are not on hormones."

Deciding to take hormones is a personal decision. The research data, while reassuring, is not yet definitive, although at this point even the most conservative experts are confident that low replacement doses of estrogen are safe when taken for up to eight years. Women with high risk factors for developing breast cancer may want to be considerably more cautious, however. You will have to balance your current level of physical discomfort with your future peace of mind. If you are so afraid of cancer that taking hormones would keep you in constant anxiety, you should respect your feelings. But if you have been avoiding hormones because of unfounded fears, this information may help you put things in perspective.

Whether or not you decide to take hormones, there are some things you can do to prevent breast cancer. While recent research indicates that fat intake may not affect the development of breast cancer, heavy alcohol consumption shows modest but significant associations with its development. So cut down on your consumption of alcohol. No particular alcoholic beverage seems to be more responsible than any other.

Also, increase your fiber intake. Fresh vegetables, fruits, and whole grains are good sources of fiber. Mounting evidence indicates that dietary fiber affords protection against breast cancer. Finally, keep at a minimum your consumption of smoked, salt-cured, charcoal-cooked, and nitrate-preserved foods.

Since most cases of breast cancer occur after age forty, it is essential that you give yourself regular breast self-examinations. In the shower or bath or while lying in bed at night, lift each arm and palpate the entire breast, including the underarm area. Look for any dimpling, bulging, or puckering of the skin and feel for any hard, pealike cysts. Expect some normal lumps, but let your physician check these out. In this way you will learn about the structure of your own breasts.

In addition to regular self-exams, it is also considered important to have yearly mammograms after age fifty. Unfortunately, mammograms are not infallible and some malignancies are missed. For additional protection, have your physician examine your breasts when you go for your annual Pap smear.

BREAST CANCER SURVIVORS

Chemothereapy can throw younger women into a temporary menopause, and older, not yet menopausal, women into menopause permanently. This is because chemotherapy can completely wipe out the ovaries and, in some cases, even impair the adrenal glands; estrogen and testosterone production are affected, and the decrease in hormones can be sudden and dramatic, sending receptors screaming. The result can be an abrupt menopause replete with intense hot flashes, extreme mood swings, and a precipitous drop in sexual desire, sexual arousal, and orgasm. Tomoxifin, an antiestrogen, can produce many of these symptoms as well. When you add this to the psychological impact of having a potentially fatal disease, the possible loss of a breast, and other psychological issues, it may become difficult for a breast cancer survivor to determine whether her emotional and sexual symptoms are psychologically or hormonally induced.

If you have had an estrogen-dependent cancer and as

the result of the treatment are having severe menopausal symptoms, solutions are available, but all approaches seem to be highly controversial. One of the most hotly debated subjects is the use of estrogen for women who have had an estrogen-dependent breast cancer. Some physicians feel that you are never cured of the disease and that a woman who has had an estrogen-dependent cancer is always at risk and therefore should never be put on estrogen. Others claim the complete opposite, that estrogen has no effect on breast cancer. Justification for this second point of view comes from studies on pregnancy or HRT with breast-cancer survivors. During pregnancy, a woman's estrogen levels rise 100–500 times the nonpregnant level. Yet women whose breast cancers were diagnosed while they were pregnant or those who became pregnant *after* being treated for breast cancer had the same survival and recurrence rates as women who were not pregnant at the time or did not later become pregnant. Other studies found that women taking hormone replacement therapy following breast cancer showed no significantly increased risk of a recurrence of breast cancer when compared to women not on HRT. A recent study conducted in Australia by Dr. John A. Eden indicated that women taking estrogen accompanied by a high daily dose of progestin (50 mg.) actually showed an improved survival and recurrence rate when compared to women who were not treated with hormones.

Because estrogen's effect on breast cancer is such a life-and-death concern, many women are demanding more conclusive evidence before looking to estrogen for symptom alleviation. However, when symptoms are significantly compromising a woman's quality of life, it is reassuring to know that hormone replacement therapy may not be totally out of the question.

Meanwhile non-hormone medical alternatives exist, although the professionals I interviewed disagreed as to their effectiveness. For emotional instability, physicians recommend Prozac and Zoloft. Cloridine, Aldomet, and betablockers can be used to control hot flashes. However, all of these drugs have potential side effects, so it is important to discuss each thoroughly with your physician.

A progestin such as Provera also diminishes hot flashes in about 50 percent of women. Those who get headaches on Provera may find Megace provides the same symptomatic relief without causing the headaches. Androgens control hot flashes in 50 percent of women while offering the benefit of increased libido and feelings of well-being. And don't forget that 400–800 international units of vitamin E alleviate hot flashes for some women.

In addition to Replens, vitamin E oil, chasteberry, 1–2 percent testosterone cream, natural progesterone cream, and very small doses of estrogen cream, there is a product called Vagifem made by Nova Pharmaceutical in Denmark that relieves painful intercourse and is apparently safe for women who have had breast cancer. Dr. Helen Singer Kaplan says, "Vagifem is a low-dose, local estrogen that comes in a resin that releases the molecules so slowly that it stays in the vagina. You can give it to cancer patients because the estrogen does not spill into the bloodstream. You insert a tablet in the vagina twice a week. It is not yet available in this country, but it is not illegal, so if you know someone in Denmark or England, you can obtain it." (See pages 123–26 for an elaboration on solutions for painful intercourse.)

Testosterone cream, pills, or injections can be highly effective for increasing sexual desire when chemotherapy has reduced a woman's bioavailable testosterone levels. Low doses of oral or sublingual testosterone can be taken daily, and injections of testosterone can be given once every month or so. A testosterone patch, which should be thoroughly safe for breast-cancer survivors, is currently being researched. (See pages 135–39 for a more in-depth look at the safety of the various testosterone preparations.)

An encouraging drug on the horizon for breast-cancer survivors is ORG OD 14, which is made by Organon in Denmark, where it is being used for birth control and menopausal replacement therapy. According to Dr. Ronald Young, "ORG OD 14 is a unique steroidlike drug that has the properties of estrogen, androgen, and progesterone, but does not actually contain these hormones. It was kept out of America because of a fear that it would have a negative effect on lipids. I'm working on opening it up for use here because it could potentially address the entire complex of menopausal symptoms."

Acupuncture and homeopathic remedies appear to be safe for breast-cancer survivors, but there is no real research on their effectiveness for this population of women, so you may have to experiment to see what works. Given all the controversy about estrogens, it remains to be seen whether herbs containing phytoestrogens, the estrogens extracted from plants (for example, Dong Quai and black cohosh) are safe for breast-cancer survivors. If you are concerned about using estrogen, you should probably also be concerned about using herbs containing phytoestrogens.

LIFETIME DECISION?

Many women fear that if they begin taking hormones, they will be stuck taking them for the rest of their lives, but this is not the case. You can stop HRT at any time—after taking two pills or after ten years. Or you can take them until the day you die. But do not begin taking hormones without careful consideration. Some women experience uncomfortable symptoms for a period of time after they stop taking them.

If you do decide to discontinue taking hormones, it is essential to taper off slowly. If you stop taking them abruptly, you are creating a kind of artificial menopause and the discomforts of hot flashes, insomnia, anxiety, mood swings, etc., which you had before are likely to return, sometimes with even greater intensity for a while.

"When all the things in my life finally settled down, I went off the hormones cold turkey. I had a month of horrendous hot flashes, but my periods quit soon after that and then the hot flashes stopped."

"I wasn't having particularly bad symptoms when I started on the hormones so I wasn't prepared for my reaction when I stopped them. Within a few days, I was having such intense anxiety attacks I was afraid I would have to be hospitalized."

Basically, the more slowly you reduce your estrogen intake, the fewer symptoms you are likely to experience.

"I gradually went off of Premarin and Provera over a three-month period. I took a pill every other day and then every third day and the last month I took about five estrogen pills and one Provera and I was fine for about two months. But then the hot flashes started up again."

Symptoms occur when receptors are deprived of estrogen. When you reduce your dose of estrogen slowly, you are cutting off the estrogen from only a small number of receptors at a time, so the symptoms are not likely to be as acute, although you may still have some.

* * *

There is no question that HRT or estrogen supplementation can relieve hot flashes, insomnia, painful intercourse, mood swings, irritability, and other symptoms for a woman whose daily life is being compromised to a significant degree. However, continued menstrual periods, a possible low increase in breast-cancer rate, and potential difficulty in adapting to the hormones—with negative side effects ranging from sore breasts, various allergies, and painful menstruation to serious depression—are drawbacks that need to be considered.

There is no one type of menopause and no one type of woman. Therefore, there is no one perfect treatment approach. As more products arrive on the market and more research is done, we have a greater number of options available. Consequently, locating a knowledgeable specialist to work with you, one who is abreast of the latest techniques, is essential.

Further Information

Winnifred B. Cutler, Ph.D., and Celsó-Ramon García, M.D. *Menopause: A Guide for Women and the Men Who Love Them.* New York: W. W. Norton, 1992.

Patricia T. Kelly, Ph.D. *Understanding Breast Cancer.* Philadelphia: Temple University Press, 1992.

Wulf H. Utian, M.D., Ph.D., and Ruth S. Jacobowitz. *Managing Your Menopause.* New York: Prentice Hall Press, 1990.

TO FIND A PHYSICIAN:
North American Menopause Society
2074 Abington Road
Cleveland, OH 44106
(216) 844-3334

Natural progesterone, estrogen, and/or testosterone
preparations:

Bajamar Women's Health Care
(314) 997-3414
(800) 255-8025

Belmar Pharmacy
(800) 525-9473

Bezwecken Women's Health Care Products
(800) 743-2256

Delk Pharmacy
(615) 388-3952

Snyder-Mark Drugs
(708) 529-3400
(800) 776-4378

Women's International Pharmacy
(608) 222-1911
(800) 279-5708

9

A Focus
on Alternatives:
Homeopathy,
Acupuncture,
and Herbs

For almost all *symptoms* of The Pause, effective alternative treatments to hormone supplementation and hormone replacement therapy are available. I interviewed many women who reported being helped by homeopathy, acupuncture, and herbs for problems including heavy bleeding, irritability, headaches, and hot flashes. While nothing works for everyone, these alternatives can be a boon for women who are having a difficult time physically, but who should not take hormones, have not responded well to hormones, or simply don't like the idea of taking them.

"I had terrible bleeding. I took Provera for fifteen days in the middle of the month, which was supposed to control the cycle, but I had terrible symptoms. I felt like I was pregnant. I put on five to seven pounds in those two weeks and I felt terribly depressed. My body felt awful. Then I took this homeopathic remedy called Caulophyllum. When I get my period, I take five pills every hour until the bleeding diminishes. It usually takes about five hours, but the Caulophyllum does suppress it."

Homeopathy and acupuncture tend to treat the whole person as opposed to specific symptoms. This chapter presents information about these often unknown or little-understood alternatives to the traditional hormone supplementation or replacement route.

HOMEOPATHY

Homeopathy was founded by Dr. Samuel Hahnemann, a medical doctor, in Germany in the late 1700s, and today it is quite popular in Europe. For example, 50 percent of French doctors and 45 percent of Dutch doctors consider homeopathic medicines effective, and 42 percent of British doctors refer their patients to homeopaths. It wasn't until the early 1800s that homeopathy was introduced in America.

Homeopathy views symptoms as defenses, attempts by the body to adapt to stress or infection. Consequently, to a homeopath, menopausal symptoms signify the body's effort to heal itself from the hormonal changes it is undergoing.

Homeopaths follow "the wisdom" of the body—prescribing remedies that consist of microdoses of various substances that if given in large doses to a well person would produce the precise symptoms that the patient is experiencing. This is called the law of similars. For example, Allium cepa is derived from onions. It is used for treating colds and hay fever when the symptoms are red and tearing eyes and runny nose—the same symptoms most people get when they chop raw onions.

In conventional medicine, allergy treatments borrow from this homeopathic principle, using a little hair of the dog that bit you, so to speak. The patient receives a minuscule injection of the substances that she is allergic to, so that she can acclimate to the substance and reduce her sensitivity to it. Instead of injections, however, a homeopathic remedy consists of tiny pills (or drops) that are placed under the tongue and absorbed through the mucous membranes. It is recommended that you avoid touching the pills with your hands before placing them under the tongue, because the salt on the skin can alter their potency.

The process of making a homeopathic remedy or medicine is called potentization. This is a procedure whereby one part of the substance being used is diluted with ninety-nine parts of water or ethyl alcohol and then is shaken vigorously. One part of this new mixture is further diluted with ninety-nine parts of water or ethyl alcohol and shaken again. This process is repeated, with the paradoxical result of strengthening the effect of the medicine with each dilution. A remedy diluted 1,000 times will be far stronger than one diluted only 3 times. Regardless of the substance being used, whether a plant, an herb, a mineral such as copper, or a substance obtained from the fluids of an animal, it is this process of dilution that makes the medicine homeopathic.

According to Dana Ullman, M.P.H., coauthor of *Everybody's Guide to Homeopathic Medicines*, "We don't fully understand how these small doses work. However, what we may be seeing is a resonating effect in the body much like playing a 'C' note on one piano which causes the same note on a second piano across the room to resonate. In this way, the body becomes hypersensitive and 'resonates' to the effect of the homeopathic medicine."

Homeopaths see the body and mind as inseparable. For example, because of their different genetic and emotional predispositions, three women undergoing the same work stress will not respond identically. One might react with high blood pressure, the second with an ulcer, and the third with rage and emotional outbursts. To determine the proper remedy, homeopathy looks at the woman as a whole, not just her insomnia, but her personality, food cravings, and other characteristics.

Unfortunately, because of lack of funding, alternative approaches to healing have been less rigorously researched than traditional Western medicine. However, the *British Medical Journal* reviewed 107 studies conducted between 1966 and 1990 in which homeopathic medicines were used. The results showed a positive effect by the remedies in 77 percent of the studies. Of the 16 most methodologically rigid studies, 88 percent showed the value of homeopathic intervention.

While a large number of homeopaths are medical doctors and all must be licensed medical practitioners of one type or another (nurse, acupuncturist, etc.), no specific additional training is required for a practitioner to prescribe homeopathic remedies. The National Center for Homeopathy and Homeopathic Educational Services offer directories of licensed health professionals who practice homeopathy (see "Further Information" at the end of this chapter).

Homeopathy rarely produces any lasting negative effects, but an unknowledgeable practitioner can disappoint you and waste your time and money. Before your first appointment, ask the homeopath about his or her experience, training, and history of success in treating women with your symptoms.

There are two kinds of homeopathic remedies. One, a constitutional remedy, treats the entire person. This includes not only the physical symptoms, but psychological and personality variables as well. A second type of remedy is more like a Band-Aid and is symptom-specific.

Out of a number of interviews with leading homeopaths, I have distilled a few of the constitutional remedies most commonly prescribed during The Pause. While few women will have *all* of the symptoms typical for a particular remedy, the homeopath looks for the general psychological and physical manifestations of the woman that fit a particular homeopathic medicine.

Many of these remedies are available in health-food stores, but do not treat yourself. It takes a knowledgeable homeopath to determine the correct remedy, appropriate dose, and frequency of administration.

Sepia

Sepia, made from the inky juice of the cuttlefish, is one of the remedies most often given to women during The Pause. Common symptoms for the woman who can benefit from Sepia are pimples, liver spots, dry mouth, dry eyes, and dry vagina. She is likely to feel cold, especially in her hands and feet, and apt to have low thyroid, low blood pressure, and low adrenal functioning. She feels better after exercise and seems to need it. Often she is uninterested in sex or doesn't enjoy it. She may feel nauseated, especially in the morning. She may have a sensation of bearing down in the pelvic region, and commonly has a weak back. She may be overdriven, tired, and irritable. At times, she can be snappish and would often rather be left alone.

"If a woman with these characteristics takes Sepia, it can return equilibrium to her system," reports Dr. Ifeoma Ikenze, a homeopath and physician trained at Albert Einstein College of Medicine who practices in Marin County, California. "Within a couple of months, she is likely to be a lot happier as well as getting along a lot better with coworkers and with her husband."

"I was having all those mood swings and irritability and heavy periods, and was I ever exhausted. I had warm flashes at night and I couldn't get back to sleep. I felt tired for as much as two weeks out of the month. After I started taking the Sepia pills, I had more energy for work and to live my life. It's been like a miracle, really."

Nux Vomica

Nux vomica is derived from the poison nut. Women who can be helped by Nux vomica may experience backaches, nausea, constipation, and frequent awakenings. An uncharacteristic tendency to overdo everything and drive themselves to achieve perfection may become problematic at this time. Women who can benefit from Nux vomica may also find themselves harboring a lot of anger, which can give rise to symptoms. Nux vomica is often used in conjunction with Sepia.

Natrum Muriaticum

Natrum muriaticum is made from sea salt and can restore the natural balance for the woman who finds herself becoming very introverted and emotionally sensitive. She may be holding grudges and carrying around past hurts, but finding it very difficult to cry. She may spend a lot of time thinking about the way things might have been and can have tremendous difficulty with intimacy at this time in her life.

Often women who can benefit from Natrum muriaticum have difficulty expressing their sexuality and tend to experience vaginal dryness. They may lose their hair, or hair may start to grow on their face. These women tend to feel uncomfortably warm fairly easily. Their neck area is often sensitive to clothing, and headaches before, during, or after menstruation are common.

Pulsatilla

Pulsatilla is made from the windflower. In contrast to women who can benefit from Sepia or Nux vomica, women who are aided by Pulsatilla tend to feel abnormally weepy and sensitive at this point in their lives. Little things can make them happy or sad. They perceive themselves as having great difficulty being assertive. They may also have a lack of energy, very little interest in sex, and an exaggerated need for love and support.

Women who are assisted by Pulsatilla feel hot all the time and are much more comfortable outdoors. They also have a tendency to experience severe menstrual symptoms like heavy bleeding, cramps, and irregular menses.

"My hot flashes were very disruptive and I would be awakened from sleep two to four times a night. After about ten days of taking the Pulsatilla the hot flashes diminished and I was able to sleep again. After a while longer, they went away entirely."

Lachesis

Lachesis is derived from the venom of the tropical American bushmaster snake. Women who can be helped by Lachesis may be feeling uncharacteristically bossy and overbearing. They may even be given to fits of rage, particularly premenstrually. In addition, they may feel quite jealous and may experience strong feelings of sexual desire. They tend to feel hot and often have migraine headaches. Their symptoms are most often found on the left side of the body, and they are likely to feel the worst when they wake up in the morning. These women are especially sensitive to the pressure of tight clothing, particularly around the waist.

Lycopodium

Lycopodium is made from club moss. Women who are assisted by Lycopodium often suffer an unusual lack of confidence at this time. They may procrastinate and become uncharacteristically indecisive. They also tend to say they have a poor memory and a fuzzy brain. They are likely to feel worse in the morning when they wake up and then better as the day goes on, until about 4 P.M., when they crash.

> "I was exhausted, so my homeopath did a series of blood tests to see if she could find something wrong in my blood. We couldn't detect anything identifiable so she gave me another remedy: Lycopodium. And that worked."

Women who are aided by Lycopodium tend to have stomach symptoms, a lot of gas; many foods seem to disagree with them. When they need food, they need it instantly or they get shaky and irritable, sometimes to the point where they cannot function. When they develop painful symptoms such as headaches or pain in the shoulders, the pain is generally on the right side, or it will begin on the right and move to the left.

Nonconstitutional Remedies

Female Glandular is a tincture available in health-food stores that balances estrogen and progesterone, but contains no hormones. "Female Glandular brings balance to the endocrine glands: to the ovaries, the thyroid, pituitary, adrenals, and bone marrow," reports Dr. Ifeoma Ikenze. It is particularly good for women who feel sluggish, whose periods are irregular in both timing and flow, and who are experiencing hot flashes and irritability. Since Female Glandular is not a constitutional remedy, but a Band-Aid-type remedy appropriate for acute symptoms, the particular personality manifestations of the woman have no bearing. However, it can be used in addition to one of the constitutional remedies when appropriate.

> "I took Pulsatilla and Female Glandular and within about six weeks, the hot flashes stopped. I also had a kind of mood despondency that nothing in my life seemed to be causing and I haven't noticed that for quite a while either."

Besides Female Glandular, there are other formula homeopathic remedies that combine a number of substances specifically designed for treating menopause. One of the advantages of homeopathic remedies is that they are far less expensive than Western medicines. And while you may have to take them a few times a day initially, after a while you often have to take them only once every week or month.

Drawbacks

Homeopathic remedies, however, are not panaceas and they don't work for everyone.

> "I started taking Sepia for irritability, but nothing happened except I got diarrhea. Then my breasts started to get more

tender and for a longer period of time, so at the end of the second month, my homeopath switched me to Arsenicum Album. But the only thing it did was clear up the diarrhea."

"I've had terrible irritability and depression and felt totally out of sorts, like some demon had taken possession of my personality. For three weeks, I took Cilica and Female Glandular but they didn't seem to be doing anything, so my homeopath put me on Calcaria Carbonica. I took that for a month, but had the worst weekend I ever had, so now I'm going to look into estrogen."

"It may take two and, on occasion, three attempts before finding the correct remedy," according to Dana Ullman, M.P.H. "And often, when the correct remedy is given, the woman will experience a crisis or brief period of exaggerated symptoms. Usually this is a good sign, because it means the remedy is working."

"For many years I've had frequent terrible headaches. About a week after I started taking the Nux vomica, I had the worst headache I've ever had in my life. I thought I was going to die. After almost two days it lifted, but I haven't had a headache since."

It can sometimes take five to six weeks for symptom relief and three to six months for an ultimate change with homeopathic treatments, so it is important not to give up too soon. Also, some changes tend to be subtle and women don't always recognize them until they are reminded about their initial symptoms.

I will never forget my second visit to my homeopath. I had taken Sepia for a month and the intensity of my fatigue had decreased considerably. However, I was totally surprised when she asked me about the joint pain in my neck and the cold sensation I had been feeling in my fingernail. I had forgotten that they had been my constant companions for more than a year before I began the remedy.

It is also not uncommon to need more than one homeopathic remedy. A first remedy may improve your overall health, while a second is required to further the healing process. But generally, homeopathy, when effective, tends to be gentle and rather inexpensive. However, it does require you to give up coffee (even decaffeinated coffee) and products containing menthol, since they antidote the remedies.

CHINESE HERBS AND ACUPUNCTURE

Chinese medicine is an ancient form of healing that predates Western medicine by about two thousand years. In the United States, practitioners of Chinese medicine should be state-certified, or in states without licensure, nationally board-certified. A licensed acupuncturist is required to have had a minimum of two years of academic and clinical training in acupuncture. The American Association of Acupuncture and Oriental Medicine will supply a list of acupuncturists in your state (see "Further Information" at the end of this chapter).

According to Dr. Martin L. Rossman, a medical doctor and acupuncturist in Northern California, "Acupuncture often works well for hot flashes, excessive bleeding, digestive problems, insomnia, and mood swings. But we don't know if it will have any effect on osteoporosis or heart disease."

The purpose of Chinese medicine is to harmonize the flow of energy, called Qi (pronounced "chee"), throughout the body. Some basic tenets of Chinese medical philosophy are that the amount of Qi we have depends on the amount we inherited at birth, as well as how successful we have been at protecting and maintaining this resource. According to Dr. Efrem Korngold, an acupuncturist who cowrote *Between Heaven and Earth: A Guide to Chinese Medicine*, "The kidney is the battery of the body. It stores up your reserves and enables you to cope with stress or challenges, illness or accidents."

It is possible to deplete your reserves of Qi if you exhaust yourself through overwork and inadequate rest, like most American women who hold a job, raise children, and exercise in their spare time. "Life stresses will dip into the Qi savings account," adds Harriet Beinfield, acupuncturist and coauthor of *Between Heaven and Earth*. "And when you dip into your reserves, you deplete essence, especially over the long haul. Women are particularly prone to symptoms during menopause when this depletion has caught up with them."

Most commonly, menopause signals the natural decline of kidney Qi, and menopausal symptoms are tied directly to this depletion.

Symptoms of kidney Qi deficiency are:

Fatigue
Dryness
Weakening of the eyes
Retention of water
Decline in memory and mental alertness
Loss of sexual interest
Sore back, legs, hips, or feet
Reduced menstrual flow
Sudden grayness or thinning of hair
Fragile bones or stiff joints

According to Chinese medical teachings, Qi must be replenished or at least supplemented throughout life, particularly during times of difficulty or transition when people are forced to rely on their reserves. Acupuncture, herbs, special yoga breathing exercises, sufficient rest, and healthy eating can replenish your Qi.

Korngold and Beinfield report that about 80 percent of the women they treat for menopause-related symptoms either experience a complete recovery or find their symptoms significantly diminished. If you choose to be treated by an acupuncturist, you can expect him or her to take an extensive history. As you describe your various symptoms, he or she may also watch your face for subtle colorations and listen to the sound and pitch of your voice, since both provide certain diagnostic clues. An acupuncturist may also examine your tongue and feel the pulses in both your wrists.

Chinese medicine has identified twelve pulses, each corresponding to a different organ or function. For example, the liver is responsible for many headaches, much irritability and tension, mood swings, and tightness of the neck and shoulders. Skin dryness belongs to the lung; heavy bleeding and digestive symptoms to the spleen; insomnia, hot flashes, and anxiety to the heart; and fatigue and loss of libido to the kidney. So herbs that particularly target the affected organ system can dramatically alleviate the symptoms associated with that organ.

Each pulse also corresponds to one of the twelve meridians, the major channels of energy flow in the body. According to Dr. Martin L. Rossman, "Traditional Chinese medical theory says that if your Qi is sufficient and of good quality, flowing through all the meridians, then you will be healthy and free of disease. If the energy is blocked or restricted, if it is excessive or insufficient, you have an imbalance that can make you vulnerable to disease."

To intensify or calm the energy flow, to transfer energy between the meridians, or to promote the function of one of the organs, an acupuncturist will stimulate points along the appropriate meridian which, among other things, releases neurotransmitters. The points can be stimulated through insertion of very fine needles under the skin at the appropriate spot. Needles come in individually sterilized packets to ensure that you will not contract hepatitis or AIDS. Some acupuncturists, however, use electrical stimulation, and others massage the appropriate points manually. A slow-burning herb called moxa (Chinese mugwort) is often used to heat the acupuncture point and intensify the process.

Acupuncture treatments are usually given twice a week for a few weeks. If there is a positive response, treatment can be reduced to once a week and then to twice a month, and can take place less and less frequently as the patient progresses.

Herbs are often prescribed to assist the healing process. They can help foster positive changes so that the patient requires fewer acupuncture treatments. Herbs, in their natural dried form, can be made into teas. They can also be taken in precombined formulas in a liquid extract made with alcohol and water. When a number of drops are placed under the tongue, the extracts are absorbed through the mucous membranes. If you don't want to absorb the alcohol, you can mix the extract with boiling water, which evaporates the alcohol, and then drink it as a tea.

Chinese herbs are usually combined in formulas to enhance and balance the individual ingredients. They also can be customized to a woman's particular needs and conditions.

"I had debilitating hot flashes. They just drained my energy for about four months and then my back went out and I just couldn't cope. I went on the estrogen patch, but I had a ghastly response to it—either I almost fainted when I got up or my heart was racing. I felt perfectly terrible so I went off the patch, but since nobody told me to go off slowly, I had an awful rebound effect and my hot flashes were even worse. So I went to an acupuncturist who gave me two bottles of liquid herbs. After four to six weeks my hot flashes were dramatically reduced."

In addition to resolving physical symptoms, Chinese herbs can be useful in combating mood swings, depression, and the volatile anger that can bubble up with hormonal changes. Herbs can be used at any time in life as a preventive therapy, to strengthen the body's resources and assure a smoother transition through The Pause.

Just because herbs are natural does not mean they are only benign. They can be very powerful. Taking the wrong herb or an incorrect dose can exacerbate symptoms or worsen your health. Consequently, while you can purchase many Chinese herbal formulas at health-food stores, you should take them only while under the care of an acupuncturist or Chinese medical doctor.

By the time I saw Julie Freiberg, an acupuncturist and nurse-practitioner who specializes in treating menopausal discomforts, most of my symptoms had been relieved through homeopathy. However, I was still extremely irritable and even anxious at times, and I was less energetic than I would have liked. According to Freiberg, I had an excess of liver Qi. Acupuncturists apparently find liver Qi congestion a common pattern among American women. Dr. Martin L. Rossman reports, "Liver Qi congestion is a pattern typical of the Supermom. The liver is not only important in regulating menstruation, it is also the organ responsible for the quality of organization in life. It is adversely affected by the stress of trying to accomplish too much in too little time."

To deal with this liver Qi congestion pattern, I was treated with needles for eight sessions and took a Chinese herbal formula. I took the herbs for about eighteen months, and it controlled my irritability. Once when I was on vacation, I ran out of the herbs and the old irritability returned. I had forgotten how awful it was.

Dong Quai and ginseng are other Chinese herbs often used for symptoms during menopause.

"My acupuncturist gave me Dong Quai and ginseng. They helped my mood immensely. I feel much, much better. And when I have a heavy period, which I have every three to four months, I get an acupuncture treatment and the bleeding stops."

Drawbacks

The drawback of acupuncture and herbal treatments is that they can be expensive. While some people respond positively to the first treatment, others require a longer time before they see positive results. If you decide to go the acupuncture route, you should have six to eight treatments before determining whether it is likely to be effective.

"I've been going for an acupuncture treatment once a week for six weeks now, but I almost stopped going because I got worse before I got better. Now, though, I can see the difference. I still have symptoms sometimes, but each day they get less and less."

HERBS AND PHYTOSTEROLS

In addition to Chinese herbs, I have mentioned many Western herbs throughout the book that are used to treat various menopausal symptoms. It is thought that one reason some of these herbs are effective is that they contain phytosterols, which are plant estrogens and progesterones. Plants use phytosterols for their own growth. "Using plants rich in phytosterols is remarkably different from taking hormones," says Susun S. Weed, author of *Menopausal Years*. "Phytosterols provide hormonal building blocks rather than the hormones themselves, allowing your body to create the precise amounts and combinations of the hormones needed."

Phytosterols can be obtained in a number of ways. One is through diet. Soybeans, yams, papayas, peas, and cucumbers are particularly rich in these plant hormones. The fact that the Japanese diet is so high in tofu, which is made from soybeans, possibly explains why so few Japanese women experience hot flashes during The Pause.

Herbs such as black cohosh and Dong Quai are high in phytosterols. However, according to Dr. David Shefrin, a naturopathic physician who has developed an extraction process for obtaining phytosterols, "Since phytosterols are weaker than the estrogens medical doctors prescribe, we need more of them to achieve an effect." This is why many herbalists prescribe large doses of herbs when treating menopausal symptoms. If you are taking herbs high in phytoestrogens without any progesterone, it may be necessary to obtain annual uterine biopsies or vaginal ultrasounds (if your uterine lining is thin enough) to monitor against endometrial cancer.

The major drawback to taking herbs in quantity is that it can be costly.

* * *

"I was having hot flashes and night sweats. I wanted to treat them naturally, so I took liquid Vitex for about four months and the symptoms stopped. Since I'm on the road a lot and I didn't have time to make teas, it was easier to take tinctures, even though I spent seventy dollars every two or three weeks. But I only took them for four months, so it wasn't too bad. And I'm pleased."

Phytosterols, made from special yam and soybean extracts, are available as creams that can be rubbed into the hairless areas of the body. They can also be made in sublingual form, in which tablets are dissolved under the tongue. In addition to natural progesterone, a number of pharmacies make creams and sublingual tablets that include different forms of plant estrogens and sometimes even testosterone. The use of phytosterols is still quite controversial, and current research data is slim, but we are likely to see more information coming out on these plant hormones in the next few years.

Further Information

Harriet Beinfield, L.Ac., and Efrem Korngold, L.Ac., O.M.D. *Between Heaven and Earth: A Guide to Chinese Medicine.* New York: Ballantine Books, 1991.

Stephen Cummings, F.N.P., and Dana Ullman, M.P.H. *Everybody's Guide to Homeopathic Medicines.* Los Angeles: Jeremy P. Tarcher, 1984.

Linda Ojeda, Ph.D. *Menopause Without Medicine.* Alameda, CA: Hunter House, 1989.

Dana Ullman, M.P.H. *Discovering Homeopathy: Medicine for the 21st Century.* Berkeley, CA: North Atlantic Books, 1991.

Susun S. Weed. *Menopausal Years.* Woodstock, NY: Ash Tree Publishing, 1992.

Honora Lee Wolfe. *Second Spring: A Guide to Healthy Menopause*

Through Traditional Chinese Medicine. Boulder, CO: Blue Poppy Press, 1990.

TO FIND A HOMEOPATH:

National Center for Homeopathy
801 North Fairfax #306
Alexandria, VA 22314
(703) 548–7790

Homeopathic Educational Services
2124 Kittredge Street
Berkeley, CA 94704
(510) 649–0294

TO FIND AN ACUPUNCTURIST:

AAAOM Referrals
4101 Lake Boone Trail
Suite 201
Raleigh, NC 27607–6518
(919) 787–5181

FOR CHINESE HERBAL PRODUCTS:

Roots and Legends
38 Miller Avenue
Mill Valley, CA 94941
(415) 381–5722

FOR THE HEALTH PROFESSIONAL:

Natural progesterone estrogen and/or testosterone preparations: See page 179

SECTION

III

Beyond "The Pause"

10

Ounces of Prevention: Heart Disease and Osteoporosis

A big selling point of hormone replacement therapy (HRT) is that it can diminish the chances of developing osteoporosis and heart disease. A number of women I interviewed were taking hormones to prevent bone fractures or heart attacks. However, before deciding to take powerful hormones to protect yourself against the possibility of acquiring a medical condition you do not yet have, it is important to assess your own risk of ever getting the disease. Saying every postmenopausal woman should take hormones is like saying every pregnant woman should get a Caesarean section *in case* she encounters problems during her delivery. Some women will need it. Others will not. Some women need hormones, others don't. And in addition to hormones, it is necessary to examine diet and exercise, which also play essential roles in preventing osteoporosis and heart disease.

HEART DISEASE PREVENTION

Cardiovascular disease is the number one cause of death in Western society. Black women have 1.5 times the risk of white women when it comes to dying of cardiovascular disease.

Estrogen protects the heart and the cardiovascular system. This is one of the reasons that before the age of fifty, women are six times *less* likely to have cardiovascular disease than men. But after menopause, women begin to lose this edge. Within thirty months after menopause, women's HDL (the "good" cholesterol that keeps the arteries clear of fatty deposits) begins slowly to go down and LDL (the "bad" cholesterol that causes the buildup of plaque in the arteries) rises. Women's cholesterol profiles start resembling men's, and ten years postmenopause, women's rate of heart attack escalates. So a woman who may be at low risk for heart disease at age fifty may not be at low risk once she reaches age sixty, especially if she does not improve her diet and exercise patterns.

Smoking alone accounts for 50 percent of all heart attacks. If you smoke even a few cigarettes a day, you have *doubled* your risk. Other factors significantly increase the risk of coronary vascular disease as well.

Risk factors for heart disease are:

Smoking
30 percent above ideal weight
Parent with a heart attack before age fifty-five
Hypertension
Both ovaries removed
Ratio of HDL to total cholesterol of 4.5 or higher
Physically inactive

The more of these factors you have, the higher your risk and the more helpful estrogen will be.

Hormones as Prevention

Most experts agree that estrogen therapy reduces heart attack and stroke by approximately 50 percent. The well-known Nurses Health Study that followed more than 48,000 postmenopausal women showed that women who at one time had taken estrogen had a 25 percent reduction in the risk of cardiovascular disease. There was a 50 percent reduction for women who were still taking estrogen. And there was no increased risk of stroke. Even women without the usual heart disease risk factors had a lower risk with estrogen therapy.

Estrogen seems to protect the cardiovascular system in a few ways. Generally, it lowers blood pressure. Receptors in the blood vessel walls, when stimulated with estrogen, open the blood vessels and promote good blood flow in much the same way that estrogen increases blood flow to the pelvic area and helps sexual function.

Estrogen directly affects cholesterol levels in two additional ways. As Dr. John Arpels explains, "First, estrogen *increases* receptors that inactivate the bad cholesterol (LDL) and prevent it from turning into plaque. Second, it increases the reusability of the good cholesterol (HDL) by lowering the enzyme that destroys it." Since cholesterol levels are directly related to cardiovascular disease, you can see why estrogen can be an effective preventative for those at risk.

Physicians used to think that only estrogen taken orally had a positive effect on blood lipid levels (cholesterol). But it turns out that non-oral approaches (the skin patch or tablets taken sublingually or inserted vaginally) may have a similar benefit. However, it takes about six to twelve months longer to achieve the same lowered cholesterol levels with a non-oral method, because the liver gets a constant daily dose of estrogen rather than a large initial dose in the first few hours after taking it by mouth.

Natural progesterone and nonandrogenic progestins, such as Provera, do not seem to affect blood lipid profiles negatively as much as can progestins, like Norlutate, which are made from androgens.

Because the chance of dying from a coronary is more than ten times greater than the chance of dying from breast cancer, some doctors advocate taking HRT for protection from heart disease regardless of the woman's risk of breast cancer. However, each woman's risk pattern needs to be assessed individually before she makes a decision. In the words of Dr. Meir Stampfer, a researcher at Harvard Medical School, "Unless you are at very high risk of cardiovascular disease, you can probably protect yourself adequately without hormones by changing your diet and exercise patterns. And whether or not you take hormones, if you *really* want to protect yourself, you should adjust your diet and exercise as well."

Still, there are some women who manufacture high levels of bad cholesterol (LDL) despite an impeccable diet. These women can benefit enormously from taking estrogen.

Exercise

We humans are animals, designed by nature to use our bodies. Regular *aerobic* exercise for a minimum of twenty minutes a day or sixty minutes three times a week will condition your heart and raise the level of your good (HDL) cholesterol. Research shows that as you become more physically fit, you reduce your risk of dying from either cancer or a heart attack. And a Dallas study of more than 3,000 women showed that an unfit woman could reduce her risk of dying by almost 50 percent, at every age, if she became fit (the same benefit she would derive from taking estrogen). "Active adult women may be two decades younger physiologically than sedentary women of the same chronological age," says Dr. Barbara Drinkwater of the Pacific Medical Center in Seattle. "While we can't guarantee that exercise will prolong life, it will enhance one's quality of life."

If you have not exercised in a few years, you should get a medical checkup or exercise stress test. Always stretch before exercising and then begin slowly. Gradually work out longer and with greater intensity, but don't try to build up too fast. In fact, research shows that women who progress from inactivity to *some* activity get the most help from exercise.

Choose exercises you enjoy—or could learn to enjoy. Instead of working out in a gym, you might prefer bicycling outdoors. Rather than meeting a friend for lunch, go for a walk together. Good conversation can take your mind off the physical exertion. When you do exercise alone, you might find that listening to music or books on tape keeps your mind off the effort. Some women enjoy yoga, aerobics, or samba classes. Figure out what's right for you and add regular exercise into your life. Schedule it in ink, so it won't be erased by a dental appointment or dinner party.

I go to the gym on Mondays, Wednesdays, and Fridays after I drop my daughter off at school. On Tuesdays at 8 A.M. and Thursdays at 1 P.M. I walk with friends. Until I nailed down these times, I exercised inconsistently, often canceling because I had too much work or other impressive-sounding excuses. While I *hate* to exercise early in the morning, and often feel I need more hours in a day to keep up with my projects, I truly feel *much* better after working out. In fact, I have grown to cherish this time and miss it terribly when I travel.

If we are going to preserve our health, it is essential to make time for ourselves, both for exercising and relaxing.

Diet

The Framingham Study, which researched 5,200 residents of Framingham, Massachusetts, found that in more than forty years, *not one person* with a cholesterol count of 150 milligrams per deciliter or lower had a heart attack, and the chance of heart attack rises directly with a rise in LDL cholesterol levels. So get your cholesterol levels checked regularly.

A diet low in saturated fats and cholesterol and high in fruits, vegetables, and whole grains will keep cholesterol levels low for most women. If you limit your fat intake to 30 percent or less of your calories, you typically cut your blood cholesterol level by 10 to 15 percent. Try to stick to polyunsaturated fats like safflower oil, soybean oil, sunflower oil, sesame oil, corn oil, canola oil, and soft margarine. Avoid saturated fats, found in red meats, lard, butter, full-fat dairy products, and foods containing shortening, palm oil, coconut oil, and hydrogenated oils.

Learn to substitute nonfat for high-fat items. Use lemon juice, chicken broth, wine, or vinegar instead of butter and oils. Substitute nonfat yogurt for sour cream or mayonnaise and select ricotta cheese or Neufchâtel instead of cream cheese. Choose part-skim cheeses such as farmer's, mozzarella, lappi, hoop, and Jarlsberg.

Substitute dried beans, peas, and other legumes for meat. If you do eat meat, make sure it is lean, and trim the fat before cooking. Be sure to drain the fat during and after roasting, baking, or broiling. And never fry your food. Eat skinless poultry and only nonfat dairy products. Avoid organ meats, egg yolks, sausages, and hot dogs, which are high in cholesterol, and nuts, peanut butter, olives, and avocados—which are all high in fat. A low-salt diet is important if you want to reduce high blood pressure.

Avoid	*Increase*
Coconut	Fruits
Whole-fat dairy products	Vegetables
Butter, ice cream	Pasta and noodles
Foods fried in	Cereals
hydrogenated oil (e.g.,	Dried beans and peas
french fries, potato	Tofu
chips, pastries)	Most breads
Most cheeses	
Mayonnaise	Allowable oils:
Poultry with skin	Olive oil
Bacon	Peanut oil
Organ meats	Safflower oil
Egg yolks	Sunflower seed oil
Tuna in oil	Corn oil
Sausage, hot dogs, cold	Soybean oil
cuts	Canola oil
Vegetable shortening	
Palm oil	
Coconut oil	
Hydrogenated vegetable	
oils	

Fiber helps to lower cholesterol levels, so make sure your diet includes foods with unprocessed fiber: raw fruits and vegetables that include their skins, bran and whole-grain products such as whole wheat bread and cereals rich in oats, corn, or wheat, as well as legumes, which include lima beans and peas. However, bear in mind that a diet *too high* in fiber seems to lower estrogen levels. As always, moderation is the key.

Vitamins

Vitamin C is necessary for cardiovascular health and to combat the effects of stress. Many researchers recommend megadoses of vitamin C—from 500 to a few thousand milligrams per day. To find out whether you are taking too much vitamin C, watch for mild diarrhea, which indicates you should lower the dose. Tablets are best. Vitamin E supplement in excess of 100 international units per day has been associated with a reduced risk of coronary disease when the supplement is taken daily for more than two years. A baby aspirin once a day is also suggested for cardiovascular protection.

OSTEOPOROSIS

Osteoporosis is a disease whose name literally means "porous bones." If enough bone mass is lost, bones become weakened and susceptible to fracture. Normally, 10 percent of the skeleton is lost and renewed each year. Osteoclasts are cells that remove old bone and are then filled in by cells called osteoblasts that create new bone. As long as osteoclasts and osteoblasts are in balance, skeletal mass remains constant.

However, lowered estrogen results in the increased reabsorption of old bone, creating more holes. At the same time, aging decreases the life span of the osteoblasts and makes them less efficient at filling in the holes. Also with age, calcium, which is necessary for bone formation, is absorbed less well through the digestive tract. The net result is that we are *all* likely to have osteoporosis to some degree. But having osteoporosis does not necessarily lead to fractures. The truth of the matter is that only a few of us will experience a fracture *because* of osteoporosis, especially with proper diet and exercise.

According to Dr. Bruce Ettinger, osteoporosis specialist at Kaiser Permanente in San Francisco, "The average Caucasian American woman has about a fifteen percent chance of suffering a hip fracture if she lives to be eighty-two. However, if she lives to be ninety, her risk goes up to thirty percent and continues to increase with age. But this increase with age has *very little to do with bone loss*. Fractures in old age are predominantly caused by loss of agility and ability to right ourselves once we have gotten off balance. Poor balance is also a side effect of many medications that are taken more frequently in older age. Hip fractures occur when we fall badly, and this can happen even when our bones are good." The major problem with hip fractures is that they are disabling and some women lose their independence as a result.

Dr. Ettinger continues, "Wrist fractures work a bit differently. Wrist fractures are believed to occur when you fall properly. You use your arm to break the fall. Unlike hip fractures, which increase with age, the risk of wrist fractures remains fairly constant after age sixty, with about a fifteen percent lifetime risk."

Statistically, a woman runs a very small chance of experiencing a fracture due to osteoporosis of the spine. The loss of height due to compression of the spine that takes place with age, and the slightly rounded back, is not generally painful or serious, and a severe curvature of the back is rare. Most women who have back pain suffer from arthritis, which presents a much greater problem for older women than osteoporosis.

These lifetime risks are still averages, so they don't say much about each of our probabilities as individuals. We are not all created equal. And we are not all equally likely to get osteoporosis. Some of us are at much greater risk than others.

Risk factors for osteoporosis are:

Smoking
Heavy drinking
High consumption of caffeinated drinks
Fair-skinned Caucasian or Asian
Thin-boned
No children
Sedentary lifestyle
Menopause completed or ovaries removed before age forty
Insufficient milk, especially between ages one and sixteen
Use of cortisone or thyroid medication
Mother, grandmother, or aunt had osteoporosis
Periods stopped for an extended time because of anorexia or bulimia

None of these risk factors alone is sufficient to predispose you to getting osteoporosis, but a combination of factors will increase your likelihood of developing the disease.

If you are concerned about your chances of developing osteoporotic problems, hospitals and special clinics have safe, modern equipment that measures bone density.

If you have a number of risk factors, you should begin measuring your bone density when you are thirty-five. If your bone density measures within the normal range, you are not at risk for osteoporosis, at least not at this time. However, since bone loss accelerates during The Pause and for about ten years afterward, you should get remeasured every couple of years to ensure that you have not started to lose bone mass too rapidly.

Hormones

Hormone replacement therapy for prevention of osteoporosis appears to apply largely to women who are at high risk because they are *already* showing a measurement of bone mass depletion that is above average for their age. The estimate is that estrogen replacement reduces the risk of fracture by 50 percent. Estrogen, either by pill or by patch, prevents the rapid acceleration of bone *loss* by the osteoclasts. This is particularly true during and after The Pause, when bone loss is most rapid. However, a recent study by Dr. Ed Lufkin, associate professor of medicine at the Mayo Clinic in Rochester, Minnesota, shows that you may be able to wait and not take estrogen until after you are already showing bone density problems. According to this study, the positive effects of estrogen were greatest in *older* women, with *documented osteoporosis*. He found an 8 percent *increase* in spine density in the first year for women using estrogen with an average increase of 15 percent over three years. The effect on the forearm and hip bone was far less dramatic, but still positive for estrogen users. "The main conclusion we drew from this study," reports Dr. Lufkin, "is that age itself is no longer a barrier to hormone treatment. Some of the patients who had the most dramatic response to treatment were women who had a greater number of fractures and were much further past the menopause."

Estrogen is also essential in order for the body to use calcium. But if you have sufficient body fat to produce the estrogen, you may have less to worry about. Here again, thin finishes last.

In addition, it appears that the most important protective function of estrogen may lie in its prevention of the age-related deterioration in reaction time. This means that if you take estrogen you may be more able to catch yourself and prevent a fall. According to Dr. Stanley Birge, director of the Program on Aging at Washington University School of Medicine in St. Louis, "The incidence of hip fractures accelerates *after* the osteoporotic process in postmenopausal women slows down. Also, wrist fractures are declining just when we see hip fractures increasing exponentially—after the age of seventy. This means women are falling badly; they are not using their arms to break their fall. Finally, estrogen only protects women from hip fractures if they are currently taking the hormone. All this, plus studies showing estrogen's positive effect on mental functioning as well as on Alzheimer's disease, leads us to the conclusion that the positive effect of estrogen is more the result of a change in the woman's reaction time and ability to fall correctly than anything to do with bone density."

If you are taking estrogen only for prevention of osteoporosis, you can cut the dose to half that of normal replacement if it is accompanied by a daily intake of 1,500 milligrams of calcium. Used with estrogen, the synthetic progestins do not diminish estrogen's effectiveness in reducing fracture risk. However, if you stop taking the estrogen, you will experience the same accelerated bone loss that would have occurred during the years following menopause had you not been taking the hormone.

It also appears that low doses of testosterone can benefit women at high risk for osteoporosis because testosterone increases bone density. Dr. Notelovitz has been studying a combination estrogen-testosterone hormone replacement therapy. He says, "Although testosterone has been reported to cause liver damage, we have seen no negative effect on the liver for the low doses we give women. However, since testosterone does have a very slight negative impact on cholesterol levels, a combination of estrogen and testosterone is an effective solution for women who are *not* at high risk for cardiovascular disease, but *are* at high risk for osteoporosis."

Finally, hormones are only one factor in a complex matrix that determines bone health. Exercise, genetics, and calcium are equally important. Let's take them one at a time.

Exercise

Exercise is absolutely essential to maintaining bone strength and density. Studies have shown that exercise not only prevents bone loss, but actually increases bone mass. Rural people who are physically active, often carrying heavy weights for long distances, have less osteoporosis. One study showed that women who exercised for one hour three times each week *increased* bone density by about 2.3 percent, while those who did not *lost* 3.3 percent. But you must continue exercising or your gains will be lost.

Take twenty minutes a day or at least one hour three times a week to do *weight-bearing* exercise. Walking, lifting, bicycle riding, Tai Chi and tennis are all weight-bearing because you are moving your body weight as you exercise. Swimming, while good for the cardiovascular system, doesn't do much to maintain bone mass because the water holds up the weight.

Genetics

All other things being equal, people of some races have denser bones to begin with or lose bone mass less rapidly over time. For example, black females are shown to have bone mass 13 percent greater than that of white females, and white women experience fractures three times as frequently. Some of this discrepancy is due to racial differences in body mass. The larger the body, the more weight you are literally "carrying around." This weight, like weight-bearing exercise, strengthens your bones. But some of this discrepancy is probably due to other, not yet understood, genetic factors.

Calcium

Keeping calcium in the bones is absolutely essential to preventing osteoporosis. However, the problem seems to lie in the *excretion* of too much calcium as opposed to insufficient consumption. What causes us to excrete calcium is high acid production. The result is a negative calcium balance—we actually lose more calcium than we are taking in.

Calcium Thieves

A number of things contribute to high levels of endogenous acid production. Certain medications, smoking, heavy alcohol use (which also leads to more frequent falls), and consumption of three or more cups of caffeinated drinks a day are all bad for your bones. *Excessive* amounts of phosphorus can diminish bone formation, so it is important to limit your intake of soft drinks and processed foods which are high in phosphorus. Too much salt also causes the kidneys to excrete more calcium.

You may be surprised to learn that eating a diet high in animal protein also contributes to a negative calcium balance. A number of studies have shown that vegetarians have higher bone density than nonvegetarians. Countries whose residents consume the highest levels of animal protein—Norway, Sweden, Denmark, New Zealand, and the United States—all have the highest level of bone fractures. Even genetic protection can be tempered by diet.

Black women who eat a high-protein diet approach the osteoporotic levels of Caucasian women with a similar diet.

On the other hand, osteoporosis is rare in Asian and African countries where the intake of animal flesh is low. And while this may have something to do with exercise—rural populations tend to get more exercise than industrialized ones—a recent study in China found a slight but significant increase in bone loss among meat-eaters when compared to vegetarians in the same community. These Chinese meat-eaters, however, ate very little meat. Had they consumed a diet as high in meat as ours, the decrease in bone mass might have been significantly greater.

It is a myth that we need to eat large amounts of animal protein to be healthy. Many Americans eat 105 to 120 grams of protein per day—more than twice what they need, according to the World Health Organization and the Food and Nutrition Board of the United States. When the protein we consume is reduced to less than 50 grams a day, we achieve a positive calcium balance.

Now, exactly how much is 50 grams of protein? One 3-ounce portion of meat, chicken, fish, or cheese contains 21 grams of protein and has approximately the same mass as a deck of playing cards. When you realize that we take in protein from a number of food sources in addition to chicken, meat, or fish during the day, you can see how easy it is to exceed the 50-gram mark and why osteoporosis is such a big problem in this country.

Calcium in Food

We not only need to make sure that calcium is not stolen from our bones, we must also make certain that we are getting enough of it in our diet. Dairy products are very high in calcium. "A study I just completed in China," explains

Dr. Jifan Hu of Cornell University, "showed that at all ages, women who ate dairy products had a significantly higher bone mass than women who ate no dairy products."

Nonfat milk is actually higher in calcium than whole milk, so you don't compromise on calcium when you choose nonfat dairy products. Besides dairy products, green leafy vegetables are an important source of calcium: collard, mustard, dandelion, and turnip greens; spinach; and chard. Broccoli and parsley are also quite high in calcium. Orange or apple juice that is fortified with calcium is another good source. In fact, one 8-ounce glass of calcium-fortified juice contains about 300 milligrams of calcium, the same as in an 8-ounce glass of milk.

Nuts are high in calcium, but they are also high in fat, so you don't want to consume too much. Blackstrap molasses is incredibly high in calcium. Two tablespoons contain 300 milligrams.

Two herbs, oatstraw and horsetail, help to keep bones strong. Oatstraw itself is high in calcium.

Calcium Supplements

Add to your diet enough supplemental calcium to total 1,200 to 1,500 milligrams per day of elemental calcium. Take care not to take *too much* calcium. More than 2,000 milligrams per day can be harmful to your kidneys. And don't take calcium supplements without consulting your physician if you have a family history of kidney stones.

When you take calcium supplements, check the label. You need to know how much *elemental* calcium is contained in each pill. You may have to search the fine print to find it. Take the calcium in two or three doses during the day. Make sure to take part of it with meals, and part at bedtime.

Calcium supplements come in a number of different

forms. Some experts believe that calcium citrate is the best supplement because it is the easiest to absorb, even though it tends to be more expensive. If you take calcium citrate in a formula that includes malic acid, the calcium will be absorbed much more efficiently, so you don't need to take as much. If calcium citrate causes stomach upset or diarrhea, try another form. But avoid dolomite or bone meal preparations; they have been found to contain heavy metals, including lead, which can be toxic.

Many calcium supplements cannot be used because they do not dissolve well in the stomach, especially since stomach acid secretion diminishes with age. To test your brand of calcium, drop a pill in a small bowl with white vinegar and stir it every few minutes. If the tablet breaks up in fifteen minutes, it will dissolve in your stomach. If the vinegar makes no impact, your stomach acids won't either.

Tums E-X Extra Strength and Rolaids Calcium Rich are among the cheapest ways to get calcium, and personally I'd rather chew than swallow pills. Be careful, however, that you *don't* take them with meals. They reduce the digestive system's ability to absorb nutrition from food. And never take calcium that contains aluminum.

Calcium Helpers

To best use calcium, you need vitamin D, vitamin K, magnesium, copper, zinc, manganese, silicon, and boron. A good multivitamin/multimineral supplement will contain these elements.

The amounts you need from all sources, not just supplements, are:

Calcium (elemental): 1,200–1,500 milligrams per day
Vitamin D: 400 international units per day

Magnesium: 150–400 international units per day

Boron: 3–5 milligrams per day

Vitamin K, copper, zinc, manganese, silicon: amounts not determined

Whether or not you take estrogen, you still need to exercise, avoid the calcium thieves, and get enough calcium and calcium helpers to maintain bone strength.

Since bone mass loss is accelerated at the beginning of The Pause and continues for approximately ten years after your last period, you should begin paying attention to changing your diet and exercise patterns as soon as you notice an alteration in your menstrual cycle. If you want to protect your daughter's bones, make sure she gets regular exercise and eats a diet high in calcium and low in animal protein in her early life. Most bone mass is attained by age eighteen. If a woman forms stronger bones to begin with, she will be losing bone from a richer source, and even with the accelerated loss of bone that occurs at menopause, she can postpone any osteoporotic problems that may develop later in life.

Further Information

John A. McDougall, M.D. *McDougall's Medicine: A Challenging Second Opinion.* Clinton, NJ: New Win Publishing, 1985.

Lila Nachtigall, M.D., and Joan R. Heilman. *Estrogen: A Complete Guide to Reversing the Effects of Menopause Using Hormone Replacement Therapy.* New York: HarperCollins, 1991.

John Robbins. *Diet for a New America.* Walpole, NH: Stillpoint Publishing, 1987.

11

Onward
and Upward

When it comes to menopause, we hear the bad news—and I certainly have presented enough of it. But there is also a lot of good news. As women go through The Pause they seem to arrive at a new place in their lives. They take themselves more seriously. They begin to interact with their partners and coworkers differently. They make major changes in their lives, equivalent to the kind I see only after months or even years of psychotherapy.

Midlife awareness combined with the physical discomforts of The Pause act as a springboard from which women catapult themselves into a rewarding new era of their lives. This era can be as profound as their college or child-rearing years. As in a good play, the final act is often the most charged, the one that ties everything together and leaves us feeling fulfilled.

But transitions are never easy, and a major one like menopause can turn our lives topsy-turvy. It forces us to look mortality in the eye, which can have a strangely liberating effect. Like someone who has suffered a life-threatening illness, we may reevalute our goals, and try to live each moment to the fullest.

"I guess you kind of savor certain moments when you realize how brief life is. Menopause has done that to me. I realize I'm getting older, but I still want to enjoy my life. Maybe if I weren't going through so many discomforts I would take it more for granted."

"Seeing my limited time span, I'm really examining to see if I'm doing what I want to do. I'm also building into my life more of what I know I want to do. I don't push myself as much, especially since I've been having physical symptoms. I still enjoy my work, but there are other things that I haven't had time to get to and now I'm getting to them."

In the process of defining what is important, women are making peace with those things they will never accomplish.

"I think of menopause as the beginning of the last third of my life and I ask myself if I want to spend the rest of my life in a race of my own creation, a race with no end. Because I keep giving myself new hurdles to jump over. So now I'm taking one class instead of three. I don't want to lock myself into the kind of work schedule that I've done before. I want free time to read books, enjoy my friends and kids, and time to be with myself."

At this point in life, women often stop worrying about what other people think and become more concerned with what *they* think.

"I can be a crazy old lady if I want to. My daughter tells me that they'll attack me if I wear this or that but I don't care."

"Now I'm enjoying the simple things in life, solitude and walks on the beach and listening to music and going to concerts with my husband—things that really matter to me. I feel truly myself."

"I don't worry about things so much. When my husband was traveling all the time, and I was left with two children, I felt that I had to do everything in the house. But now I don't. Sometimes I'll pass by a mess and say, 'I'll just pick it up tomorrow,' or whatever. I no longer put that pressure on myself."

For most women, menopause does not mark the end of their lives, but a new beginning.

"It's an exciting time because there's a lot of change. I see it as the next half, not the last half. There's a lot to look forward to and a lot of good things yet to discover. I feel calmer now than I've ever felt. I'm feeling very centered and self-satisfied. I feel very good about where I am right now."

As hormones rebalance and hot flashes abate, energy returns in a consistent way, without the ups and downs of monthly cycles. Messy periods are done with and pregnancy is no longer an issue—all of which can free us immensely.

"I've always had to be concerned about getting pregnant. And not to be concerned every month has been a delightful, wonderful thing for me. So far as feeling attractive, I feel very attractive, vital and alive. Finally the children are grown and I'm free."

"Freedom" was a term women used over and over again. Freedom from child-rearing responsibilities, freedom from the opinions of others, freedom to be themselves.

> "I feel completely liberated, a free person doing as much as I can when I want to. And I'm really enjoying life. I'm having a good time with my kids and my grandchildren. I've been through a lot of struggles, including epilepsy, but now my kids are doing well and I'm enjoying them without the responsibility. It's great."

> "I used to be a control freak, but when I went through menopause I was totally out of control. I feel grateful it happened, though, because I'm in a very different space today. I feel like I really shed a skin. I'm not the same person I was. I'm much more laid-back, lighter, and funnier. I don't care about a lot of the things I used to care about, like how the house looks, about getting things done on time—or even getting some things done at all. I feel relieved from the pressure of trying not to make mistakes—not a hundred percent of the time, but fifty-one percent. Just enough to relax."

In other cultures we see women gaining more freedom and status once they pass through menopause. Women who have been veiled during childbearing years can take off their veils; they are liberated from monthly purifying segregations. They are free to travel, to join in activities that have been prohibited, like drinking with men. Women in Tonga are freed of childbearing taboos and can eat previously forbidden foods like porcupine and monkey, and may even engage in business. Kapauku Papuan women and Chinese women become emancipated from the powers of their husbands. In Eastern Timbira, once a woman's periods have stopped, she joins in a ritual whereby she is officially accorded the respect that men have been given. Winnebago Indian women can help construct ceremonial lodges. And many native women cannot become holy women, matchmakers, or midwives until after menopause.

For example, women in Mexico, Indian women, and Cree women of western Saskatchewan must be past menopause to exercise shamanic and healing powers.

As a result of increased status and positive role changes, women of these cultures view menopause either indifferently or as a positive event in their lives. They do not approach it with the same fear and denial as women of industrial cultures, who are not rewarded for reaching this stage of life. Women of non-Western cultures also seem to have fewer physical symptoms with menopause. Of course, genetics, stress, and diet also play a role, but when we look at most cross-cultural studies, we see that while women of other cultures appear to have many of the same physical symptoms Western women have, fewer report being bothered by them. In these non-Western cultures the positive benefits of menopause outweigh the negative. It is like the pain of first intercourse—you have a feeling that the pleasure to be derived will offset the initial discomfort.

For Mohawk women, this period of transition relates to the concept of time, time *for her,* and time spent meaningfully *on her.* Women I interviewed who were feeling best about their lives believed they had earned the right to their moment in the sun.

"I've made new goals, I want to travel, to investigate, to learn new things. There is so much out there to do and learn, but I haven't been able to take advantage of it because my family has always come first. Now my goals have become selfish again."

"It's the beginning of a new part of my life, of the part of really just being myself and taking care of me. I've been a musician all my life. Well, two years ago I took up the harp and I'm now playing for weddings and parties. I also just rented this apartment. I can do exactly what I want here and I don't have to worry about anybody."

"Wait a second. I deserve something. I've been going through all this stuff and I need to take care of me or I'll come out a rag. I need some recognition and if others aren't going to put my needs first, I will."

"I've remodeled my house. I got a new bed, a wonderful quilt, a new carpet. I am making my home mine. I couldn't have done that when I was younger. Not because I didn't have the money, but it wasn't in keeping with how I saw myself. I didn't want to spend money on myself. Now I will take facials once a month. I am really honoring myself in a different way."

One of the biggest changes I saw in my interviews was that women's attention had shifted from those around them to themselves. They no longer thought they had to be the caretakers. They no longer had to subjugate their needs to those of spouse and children.

"I have definitely come to a time when I'm not the least bit interested in putting up with my husband's foul moods or his temper or any of the rest of the stuff that he wants to use as intimidation methods. That is crap and he can just knock it off right now, because I choose not to deal with it. I have made that terrifically clear. I have become more verbal and without fear that he might decide to walk out. It's like, let me help you pack because if that's how you choose to be, you can live in an apartment by yourself."

"I have pretty much catered to everybody else. I seldom spent time with myself, doing things for myself, not even spending money on myself. I did it for everyone else, and I have a large family. I decided that I wasn't going to do this anymore and I let them all know that things would be different. They attributed it to mood swings and hot flashes and figured I'd eventually come out of it. But now things are going to be done for me. One of my daughters recognizes this and soon the others will wake up to reality."

Women not only make changes *within* their relationships; some who feel their needs are not being met terminate their relationships at this time.

"At forty-seven, just when I was going through menopause, I realized he wasn't going to marry me, we'd never get a bigger place, and with our different schedules it was totally ridiculous. I realized I had been unhappy for ten years, and had compromised myself enough. I felt, it's time for him to do a little more. And when he wouldn't, I asked him to move out."

"My lover and I were living together and I was feeling trapped. I broke up with her about a month ago. Now I want to do exactly what I want to do, every minute that I can."

Many women who are no longer in intimate relationships are becoming consciously aware of the advantages of not entering another one.

"I don't want to get involved with somebody. I'm fifty. I don't want someone sixty-five that I have to take care of if he gets sick. I'm not interested in doing that. I don't want another man in my life. I don't want to focus in on his needs or our needs. I've had it. I just want to focus in on my needs."

With or without a partner, women discover their lives opening up in new and rewarding ways.

"I have some Indian blood. I was indoctrinated into Grandmother Lodge, which you can do after your periods have stopped. They call us Gray Hairs. Something happened at that time, and since then I've been reenergized. I've always been a teacher and counselor but I've noticed a new joy and ease with my work and my life. I'm teaching in a clearer, more mature way now."

With less concern about pleasing others and more of a desire to fulfill their own needs, women often develop a new sense of authority after menopause. They begin to feel clearer, surer of who they are, more powerful.

"I feel very effective, competent, sure of myself now. I feel I have an increased sense of power. More so than ever before in my life."

Androgens, the male hormone, may play a role in increased self-assurance and assertiveness. Not only do androgen levels increase in some women, during and after The Pause, but without high estrogen levels to counter them, androgens find more expression at this time. In one study, researchers found that women developed stronger feelings of assertiveness and mastery once they had completed menopause. Many women return to school, change careers, become active in a spiritual way, or take on new creative projects.

"I had never written anything before, but over the last year I've written articles, short stories, and reviews of a couple of books and a film. And they've all been published."

"I'm single and I just started a new profession. In my first life, I was a mother. Then I went back to school and now I'm licensed as a physical therapist. So it's an adventure. And I'm traveling. I went to Japan last year and I'm going to Thailand this summer. I really like where I am right now."

"When I was fifty, as a birthday present, I started Jungian analysis because I wanted to explore this new opening in my life."

"Now I'm involving myself in politics, something I've always wanted to do before, but didn't have the time because my children always needed me."

"I've started to take my art seriously. I'm painting three to four hours a day and I'm taking classes."

Some of us even allow ourselves to show our wisdom without feeling embarrassed or apologetic.

"Someone just called me and said, 'You were recommended to me because I really want a *senior* therapist.' So I'm not freaking out about getting older."

"I've gone through a mental shift. I've entered a place where I can think of myself as being wiser. And I'm appreciating these years as the first in a new phase of my life."

Recent research shows a strong correlation between satisfying work and personal fulfillment during this stage of life. But not all women are able to move ahead with ease. Some feel trapped in their caretaking role, especially if they have ailing parents. Others don't feel the self-confidence to take the necessary steps to discover new facets of their being. Some who have recently lost a partner may feel bewildered and disoriented, even if the relationship had been less than satisfying. For these women, difficult personal work lies ahead if they are to navigate this phase of their lives successfully.

For those of you who never left the security of your homes, striking out may be a fearsome prospect. If you have dedicated your life to others, you may not be well versed at doing things for yourself. You may know how to give but not feel you have the inner strength or skills to make it on your own. If this is your situation, begin with small steps. "Start by taking one minute a day to do something you enjoy," advises Joyce A. Venis, R.N.C., a psychiatric nurse in New Jersey who runs PMS and menopause support groups. "If you don't know what that might be, experiment. Take a bath in the afternoon, work in the garden, take up a sport or form of exercise. A simple book titled *One Minute for Myself: How to Manage Your Most Valuable Asset* will help you discover what you might enjoy. If you are nursing a loved one, or are under stress, it is particularly important to find ways to take time for yourself. When you take better care of yourself, you can be more nurturing to others."

You might consider volunteering your time to an organization that could use your hands, your eyes, your lasagna. In this way, you will still be giving—but also learning new skills, making new relationships, having new experiences. For many women, volunteering is a path to developing the satisfaction that is missing in their lives.

This "third third" of your life can be a time of taking risks and doing things quite differently. Expect uncertainty and doubt to be your companions for a while. When you try new things, you might imagine that you are a researcher looking at life with no expectations in mind. Your only goal is to make a true unbiased discovery: to learn about what you enjoy doing and what you can do well. With no preconceived notions, you may find direction opening up for you in unexpected ways.

You may have to let go not only of preconceived ideas, but also of people or of jobs. One woman lost her job of twelve years and was devastated. She thought no one would want her at her age, a real problem in today's marketplace, which often values youth and sex appeal above experience and maturity. But she picked herself up, went out on interviews, and found a part-time job that paid as well as her previous full-time one. Another woman, who had recently remarried a man ten years her junior, was devastated when he decided to leave her for another woman just as she turned fifty.

"It's taken me almost two years to get over him. Even though it was clear that he didn't want me anymore, I had a hard time letting go. And it's scary to be alone. But now I'm doing volunteer work. I've taken up the piano again, and music has become the love of my life. And I've moved into a new apartment. It's like the phoenix rising out of the ashes."

Just when you want to be more on your own, you may find it difficult to disappoint your partner, who may be embarking on retirement and desirous of spending more time together. You may be winding up while your partner is winding down. Relationships can suffer from this difference in timing until a new equilibrium is worked out.

"I want to make every day count, to be exciting. My poor husband. He's not the same. He's slowing down. He wants to read a book and I want to go dancing. So we're having conflict about this at the moment."

You may want to consider forming a women's support group to help you through this period. Without support during this transition time, many women feel lost.

"I was the first one of all of our friends to start menopause and there was nobody to talk to. I felt isolated and alone out there. I would have liked to know what other women were experiencing because for a while there, I really did think I was going crazy. It was really hard to do it without support."

In the 1970s women's groups helped many of us negotiate our transitions from helpless, passive females to asser-

tive and full participants in life. We compared lives, shared our problems, and offered solutions from which other group members could partake as they chose. Rewriting our roles today, during this stage of life—as we did in the seventies—is easier with the support of other women.

"I had less anxiety because of the support group. I saw the incredible variations, that there's not one track to menopause. I also felt reassured that I'm pretty normal for what should be happening given the vast variety."

"It's really wonderful to have picked up parts of women's stories that are similar to mine. It's just made a world of difference, knowing that I'm not alone because it's been very rough, these eleven years. I could say I've been to hell and back more than once. But I've survived and my kids survived. It's like going to a twelve-step meeting; you never heard your story before, and all of a sudden someone says something, and it's like, 'My God, I'm okay. I'm all right.' "

"Being in a menopause group and listening to other women and seeing the way they took charge of their own health care helped me. Though I'm married to a physician, I had been guilty of being very passive about my health care. I've always believed that my body would take care of itself, but it turned out that I had a fibroid tumor equivalent to being twelve weeks pregnant. By the time I came to the group, I was desperate, but toughing it out. Every month I would just try to get through the four to five days of cramping and heavy bleeding. But it really took its toll. From listening to others I realized it *was* a real problem and I *wasn't* getting the right care. As a result, I've now gotten proper treatment."

According to Frederika Ebel-Riehl, coordinator of education for the Women's Health Center in Flemington, New Jersey, "The support is very important in making women realize that they are not alone. The groups empower women to make new goals, pursue a hobby, or change a career. It gets them involved and helps them concentrate on themselves and less on their roles as caretaker or even victim. I see women who had been hanging on to deadwood go back to school, start to make new friends, and identify other women as valuable sources of support."

Knowing that you are okay and on track can dissipate the feelings of uncertainty and anxiety that often accompany The Pause. One Norwegian study showed that women with a strong social network suffered fewer psychological symptoms during menopause. Another study showed that information and reassurance were sufficient in terms of easing concerns for 40 percent of women seeking help at menopause clinics.

If you want to join a support group but can't find one in your community, consider starting your own. Gather your friends and have them invite *their* friends. Limit the group to ten or twelve members. That's not too many to begin with and allows a few to drop out without leaving the group too small.

For the first two or three sessions, talk about your experiences with The Pause—both physical and psychological. Every two or three sessions, invite a guest speaker. If you each contribute $5 or so per session, you will be able to pay your expert. Even though public speaking is good for business, experts still feel more appreciated when they are financially rewarded.

Pick professionals who specialize in menopause. In this way you not only get the most up-to-date information, but you also encourage professionals to expand their interest in this area. Don't pick someone just because he or she is your gynecologist, or because you like him or her. A physician who specializes in obstetrics may not be up to date on the most recent menopause treatment protocols. For the same reasons, pick an acupuncturist, an herbalist, a homeopath, and a therapist who are experienced in working with women going through The Pause.

Use the support of the group to go out and educate those around you. Some women are reluctant to let their coworkers know about any difficulties they may be having as they go through The Pause, for fear of losing their jobs. But everyone goes through stressful transitions in his or her life. We get married, divorced, have a loved one who gets ill or dies, and we all require the support of our colleagues during these times. If we need more, we can seek professional assistance to ensure that uncomfortable symptoms do not prevent us from doing our job—whether it is mothering or manufacturing.

The more we talk to others, the more we bring menopause out of the closet. People with gay and lesbian friends and coworkers are not frightened of homosexuality. It is only when hidden in secrecy that it becomes something to be feared. The same is true of menopause. Our culture needs education about menopause. And no one is going to do it for us. It is our job. We alone can create a new image, one that projects how *we* feel about ourselves during this stage of life rather than how others have chosen to view us. If we do it well, we will open the way for our younger sisters and daughters, just as we did with the women's movement in the late 1960s and 1970s.

We can be sexy; we can be vital; we can be productive and creative. Getting older doesn't mean we're over the hill. A fine wine gets better and better for many years before it begins to turn to vinegar. In fact, many women don't come into their own until they are past menopause.

"I feel like I'm in my prime. I get to look back at half my life and I see these patterns appearing in my relationships. I get to see what I really care about and how I can have an even more positive influence on the world around me in the future."

Clearly, the years following menopause will be different in many ways from those that preceded them, but with a healthy outlook and body, the third third can be the best third of our lives.

Further Information

A Friend Indeed (newsletter)
Box 1710
Champlain, NY 12919–1710
(514) 843–5730

Menopause News (newsletter)
2074 Union Street
San Francisco, CA 94123
(415) 567–2368

MidLife Woman (newsletter)
5129 Logan Avenue S.
Minneapolis, MN 55419–1019
(612) 925–0020

Women's Health Connection (newsletter)
(all women's hormone-related health concerns)
P.O. Box 6338
Madison, WI 53716–0338
(800) 366–6632

Via (magazine)
(a guide through menopause and beyond)
P.O. Box 3000
Denville, N.J. 07834

Elizabeth Sher
Approaching the 14th Moon Videotape.
I.V. Studios (510) 528-8004, 1993.

Men: Partners in Menopause*

If you are living with a woman going through The Pause, who feels emotionally out of control and physically unwell, you may be at your wits' end. You may even doubt that her reactions are really due to menopause. You may worry that Dr. Jekyll has turned into Ms. Hyde—permanently.

For anyone who has not gone through The Pause, it is impossible to understand fully what the experience is like. Your partner may appear healthy, but actually feel unwell either all or some of the time. She may feel emotionally flat and unmotivated. She may awaken a number of times during the night and have difficulty falling back to sleep.

*I have directed this chapter to male partners since female partners of women going through *The Pause* are more likely to read the book in its entirety, the information ultimately pertaining to them as well. However, pages 238 to 242 contain information that is not found elsewhere in the book.

She may feel uncharacteristically anxious or insecure. She may develop the infuriating habit of turning the heat on and off during the day or throwing the covers off on cold nights. Minor frustrations may enrage her or the slightest criticism destroy her.

While her transition to menopause can range anywhere from being mildly disruptive to a full-blown nightmare, remember, she'll eventually reach the other side—the process does end. This may be the most important point. Your partner will gain a new hormonal equilibrium and will begin feeling better. But the journey may be difficult, and during the transition your relationship may change.

Change, however, is not necessarily bad. While the status quo may feel comfortable, some degree of friction and conflict may inaugurate new growth. Conflict may create tension and vulnerability, but when handled well it can increase intimacy. You may learn to be more open with each other. You may each define yourselves and your needs more clearly. In the end, you may find that when your partner's hormones settle, your relationship is stronger and more balanced and has taken on dimensions that you never anticipated.

Commonly, a woman's partner may feel he is to blame when she has a difficult time with The Pause. You may worry that you have done something to cause her overly emotional response or withdrawal from the relationship. Often this is not the case. Many women are not able to control their emotions completely because fatigue and internal upheaval are playing havoc with them.

Emotional and physical symptoms can begin anywhere from two to ten or more years before a woman's periods actually stop and can last for as long as a year or two after her last menstrual cycle. During this period, as the ovaries begin to shut down, estrogen, progesterone, and often testosterone levels are changing. However, lowered levels of estrogen are primarily responsible for most nonsexual symptoms—and even for some of the sexual ones.

Every woman has an estrogen set-point, the particular level of estrogen she needs to function without symptoms. Because estrogen affects her brain and nervous system as well as numerous other bodily functions, when her estrogen level dips below her set-point, she is likely to experience emotional and physical symptoms. She may feel irritable, anxious, depressed, impatient, forgetful, or fuzzy-headed and fatigued. These emotional discomforts are likely to be compounded when the lack of estrogen also causes insomnia or hot flashes. Some women experience headaches, joint pains, gastric upset, pain with intercourse, or a lack of sexual desire. Few women will experience *all* of these symptoms, and many women have symptoms that are bothersome but not incapacitating. The symptoms can, however, be so disconcerting that nearly 40 percent of women seek medical treatment.

It might help to think of your partner as someone withdrawing from a drug. In fact, she is withdrawing from her own production of estrogen. When you stop using a drug, you experience symptoms because receptors that are dependent on that drug are being starved. If a drug is reduced gradually, symptoms are less severe, but a woman's estrogen level is not usually declining in a gradual manner. At times she may be producing plenty of estrogen; at other times, not. For example, if she ovulates particularly well, her hormones may surge. These surges of estrogen production are like fixes to a drug addict who is trying to detoxify. She cannot effectively adapt to the reduced estrogen level when it keeps getting pumped up again and again. And even in a gradual detoxification, symptoms generally appear. Deprived of estrogen, receptors in her body scream out and she suffers symptoms. After a longer period of deprivation, her receptors die off and the symptoms finally stop. However, when her estrogen levels increase, new receptors are formed—only to be deprived once again, creating more symptoms as estrogen levels inevitably decline permanently.

The woman is riding the roller coaster of her fluctuating hormones. She would rather not be so cross, so exhausted, so sensitive or enraged. These are direct reactions to decreased estrogen. And having headaches, joint pain, or breast tenderness is no fun and can readily put her in a bad mood. It is scary to feel your heart palpitating for no reason. Can you imagine the frustration and exhaustion of feeling as if your body is on fire and then bathed in sweat when you least expect it, day and night?

Some women have an easier time with menopause than others. These women are either less reactive to their changing hormonal balance or have sufficient body fat to keep their estrogen levels elevated. Estrogen is manufactured in the fat cells (as well as in some muscle and brain cells). It is in a woman's best interest to gain *some* weight as her ovaries begin producing less estrogen, and most women do gain weight during The Pause. It appears to be nature's way of helping her adapt.

Most women experience only mild to moderately distressing symptoms; about 10 to 15 percent find their symptoms debilitating. These women are not weak or neurotic, they are simply more sensitive to their shifting hormones. If your partner is being tormented by The Pause, you can encourage her to get help, not from a psychiatrist, but from an acupuncturist, homeopath, or physician experienced with treating women during this transition. You can also help her with diet and exercise, both of which can ease her symptoms.

Research shows that regular exercise increases estrogen levels and reduces hot flashes and other symptoms of The Pause. Exercise not only increases energy, it helps you sleep better and releases endorphins that elevate your mood. Exercise such as walking, jogging, and bicycle riding, during which you bear the load of your body weight, helps stem osteoporosis. Aerobic exercise significantly decreases the risk of heart disease.

The kindest thing you can do for your partner's short-term and long-term good health is encourage her to exercise. Minimum time spent exercising should be at least twenty minutes daily or one hour, three days a week. You may offer to take over some of your partner's responsibilities or chores to give her time to exercise. And when she is feeling depressed or emotionally out of sorts, you can help transform her mood by taking her hand and leading her outside for a brisk walk together. Exercising together will help both of you stay healthier and more attractive.

In addition, a diet that is good for your partner will also improve your health. A low-fat diet protects you both from heart disease. A diet that contains minimal animal flesh will also protect your bones. Low sugar consumption keeps you both trim and helps reduce her premenstrual symptoms. A reduction in dairy products will reduce her premenstrual symptoms as well.

In addition to encouraging your partner to prepare meals that follow these guidelines, you can support her dietary needs when you cook or shop. The higher her diet is in vegetables, fruits, pastas, and grains, the healthier she is likely to be. And the healthier she is, the less of your time will be required to care for her in your later years. What works for her health ultimately works best for you, no matter how you look at it. If you feel the need for more animal protein, a small portion of broiled meat, fish, or poultry could be added to the menu. But meat and poultry skin are not in the best interests of your heart either: they contain significant amounts of fat and cholesterol.

There are also some concrete things you can do to-

gether to manage your partner's emotional mood swings
more effectively. Chapter 3 discusses a number of behaviors that she can change. The following are some behaviors you can control.

First of all, tell your partner that you want her to keep
you posted as to her state of mind, like a weather report:
clear skies ahead or storm brewing. Agree that as soon as
she becomes aware that her temper is short, she is to let
you know so that you can keep your distance.

"I really appreciate it when she says, 'I'm off center, so
don't press me. If there is something you want to talk to me
about, write it down and we can talk about it later.' "

This practice of writing things down and then addressing them later can save the day. It allows you to drop the
matter at a time when your partner is really not emotionally ready for productive discussion, without losing sight of
the issue. Don't just swallow your concerns because you're
afraid to approach her. Being in The Pause doesn't give
your partner the right to jump down your throat whenever
she feels like it, but it does give her the right to have your
special consideration. Tell her to let you know when she
feels fit to discuss the checkbook overdraft or the mix-up
over who was going to pick up the kids, for example. You
may have to wait a couple of days, but agree not to postpone issues much longer than that. Like weeds, irritations
tend to grow rapidly when not attended to.

"Now when something is bothering me and she responds in
a way I think is irrational, I write it down. I don't always
give her the letter, but if I write it down, I can look at it
later and see whether I still think it's important enough to
bring up. When it doesn't seem very important once I get
some distance from it, I drop it. But other times, the issue

is a real issue and I don't want it to get buried under her barrage of emotions."

When you think your partner's response is out of proportion to the circumstances, it may be useful to mentally divide the intensity of her reaction by ten. I'm not encouraging you to dismiss her feelings or her concerns, but The Pause causes emotions to be intensified. Something that might have bothered her only slightly in the past may infuriate her today. Keep in mind that she may tend to use dynamite when a flyswatter would be sufficient.

If you can determine the real concerns behind your partner's upset, it will be more fruitful to *validate* her concerns instead of attacking her exaggerated response—for example, acknowledging that you forgot the milk rather than blasting her for making a federal case out of it. Look for the grain of truth in her words and admit to that truth, then disengage from the fray. Give her some distance so that she can try to regain her equilibrium on her own.

"Don't get hooked in. What helped me the most was when my husband stopped trying to fix me. Because when he would tell me that my hormones were going crazy or would look hurt so I would feel guilty, it would just make things more intense. When he backed off, I could turn it around for myself. He would say, 'It seems like you're having a hard day or a hard time. Is there anything I can do?' If I said, 'No, there is nothing you can do,' that would be the end of it. It was terrific."

One friend of mine was going through a prolonged and very difficult menopause and her boyfriend just couldn't figure out how to deal with it. He felt enraged, frustrated, and impotent. Finally I asked him how he would respond if she had a chronic illness and felt terrible most of the time. I suggested he read *Mainstay* by Maggie Strong,

about living with a chronically ill person. And while menopause is certainly not a lifelong infirmity, it generally
doesn't pass in a few months either.

> "Thinking of her as chronically ill was helpful to me. I
> started to realize that she wasn't doing these things volun-
> tarily, that she was having a difficult time, too. I began to
> recognize that I had needs that I wanted her to take care of,
> but she just couldn't take care of them the way I wanted her
> to at the time. It helped me give her more slack and that
> was very helpful."

Later, my friend said,

> "I almost killed him when he showed up with that book. I
> almost killed you. It infuriated me when he looked at me
> like a sick person. I can't stand to be sick. On the other
> hand, in my saner moments, I was really appreciative that
> he was trying to adjust himself to me. So that was really
> helpful."

Take the time to check in with your partner every day.
Ask her how her day went, how she is feeling both emotionally and physically. Offer your support; it really doesn't
take much. Most women find it comforting just to know
they have a supportive partner, someone willing to listen
and take their needs seriously.

I realize that you are being asked to be patient and understanding, often leaving your own needs unmet because
of your partner's preoccupations, but each partner gives
more at different times during the life cycle. You may have
given more after the birth of your child. She may have
given more at certain times during your career. However,
while your partner's biological and psychological needs are
likely to be more pressing at this time, your needs must be
addressed as well. If they are not, you will undoubtedly

find ways, if not directly, then indirectly, to express your frustration and resentment.

You may resent your partner's unavailability. As she becomes consumed by her own transformation, she may have less energy to devote to you. You may also find that she is less willing to compromise her needs in favor of yours, as she has in the past. If you are a decade or more older than your spouse, her new sense of self may be particularly distressing. With children gone, she may be looking outward while you are yearning for a quiet retirement. You may be needing more from her just when she is less emotionally available.

When you feel your own needs are getting short shrift, make sure you don't push yourself into the corner of resentment. Talk to your partner about it when she is feeling both physically well and emotionally grounded. Pick one issue and choose it carefully, so that you have the best chance of creating a positive change. Concentrating on one area is likely to be more effective than a diffused focus on a larger field. Are you longing for more physical tenderness or sexual frequency? Do you feel she is not taking your concerns about her health seriously? Do you feel demeaned by her impatience?

You don't have to come up with a solution during this first conversation. Actually, it is often more expedient to spend time defining the problem and then to go off separately to mull the situation over so that you can both come up with a few alternative solutions. Remember, you are in this together and the challenge is to come up with a solution that works for both of you.

MALE AND FEMALE LIFE CHANGES

While modern medical literature does not support a male physical transition comparable to the female menopause, it is clear that men go through a major period of re-evaluation during their mid-forties to mid-fifties. For some men, this reappraisal may be triggered by their wife's menopause. Menopause is a clear mortality marker for both of you. It signals that the autumn years are approaching, a reminder that neither of you will live forever.

Many men make major career changes at this time in an attempt to actualize their lives or fulfill their secret ambitions. A deep dissatisfaction with your own life, combined with a realization that death is no longer an abstraction, may encourage you to take certain risks at this time.

For women, the menopause marks a similar period of evaluation. Most women lose a major role at this time—they are laid off, so to speak, as their children seek independence. This is the time when a woman must evaluate her life and assess the goals she would like to fulfill before it is too late.

Both men and women often evaluate their marriages during this "menopause" period. This process can stress a relationship tremendously. It may be difficult to figure out whether the problem lies in the actions of one of the partners or is more a reaction to this internal midlife evaluation process.

Sadly, relationships can suffer the fallout from internal growth pains. Not all couples can adapt to the changing needs of one or both individuals. But some that might be able to are never given the chance. These midlife crises are so common they have become a cliché. But they are not a joke. They break up families, sometimes even destroy lives. Beware of making hasty decisions during this time.

LOVEMAKING

Menopause can affect a woman's sex life. The lack of estrogen can cause the vaginal lining to thin and become less elastic. It can also reduce lubrication significantly. The result is that intercourse becomes painful for many women. These changes can begin very early in The Pause, when a woman is in her early forties or even late thirties.

If your partner experiences pain with intercourse, she may no longer look forward to sex. She may also lose desire if her hot flashes, insomnia, and other symptoms of estrogen deprivation are so severe that they interfere with her energy and sense of well-being. None of us feels like making love when we feel ill.

Testosterone affects a woman's sexual desire in the same way it affects a man's. We don't know why, but about half of all women experience a sharp decrease in the ovarian production of testosterone around the time of menopause. For these women, sexual interest decreases. It is not that a woman is angry at her partner or has fallen out of love; her body simply is no longer aware of sexual energy. As one woman said, "I've forgotten the purpose of sex. I just can't figure out why in the world anyone would bother to do it. So I know I need to use the testosterone cream again. When I use it, it all becomes perfectly clear."

Many men have difficulty accepting that hormones can cause this decrease in sexual interest. They take it personally and feel undesirable.

"I have a hard time believing that her desire for me has to do with her hormones. I keep thinking that she should be sexually interested because of *me*."

But as biological creatures, when it comes to sex, we are ruled more by hormones than most of us would like to think.

Your partner can take supplemental testosterone if her lack of desire is caused by low testosterone. And she can take estrogen (or estrogen plus progesterone after her periods stop) if her desire has plummeted because of physical discomforts caused by diminished estrogen. She can use an estrogen cream vaginally to restore her vaginal tissues if pain with intercourse is her only complaint. Acupuncture as well as homeopathic and herbal remedies are also available.

A lubricant such as Astroglide or K-Y jelly can be used if insufficient lubrication is her sole problem. Encourage her to use a lubricant. For months intercourse had been painful for me, and I kept complaining that I was too dry. David didn't agree. The result was a recurring yeast infection. Once he realized that lack of lubrication really was the problem, he became very supportive. He not only makes sure the lubricant is accessible before we make love, but he takes care that we never run out.

Some women, however, lose sexual desire for reasons that have nothing to do with The Pause. Your partner may never have liked sex to begin with—maybe because of early sexual abuse or a puritan upbringing. Now she may finally feel legitimately freed from it. Or resentment may have dampened her sexual interest. Are you able to resolve your disagreements or does unexpressed anger hang in the air like a thick fog? Do you try to make all of the decisions in the relationship or does your partner have a voice? Sometimes a woman who feels she has no power in the relationship—power to be heard, to make decisions, to be taken seriously—has power only when she withholds. She may wield her power in the bedroom by saying "no."

How well do you think your partner is satisfied by your sexual relationship? If you have doubts, check it out with her. If your partner is not satisfied sexually, she may see no reason to participate in an activity that produces pleasure for you but discomfort for her. And just because she has not complained does not mean she is enjoying it. She may think she is protecting your ego by keeping her feelings to herself, unaware that the loss of your sex life may be more devastating than any blow to your ego.

Do you take care with your appearance? Do you dress attractively and keep your body well-toned and exercised? Do you shower and shave when sex is on your mind? And how about brushing your teeth before making love? Women are often more sensitive to smells than men. I cannot tell you the number of women who report that they are put off sexually because of their partner's offensive body or mouth odor.

Do your part to keep up the romance, both in and out of the bedroom, if you want to maintain an active sex life. Leave your partner loving notes, phone her during the day, or bring home small presents or treats to convey your affection. Tell her that you love her and that she looks good—often. Feeling loved and wanting to express it in return are major sexual incitements for women and probably some of what attracted her to you in the first place.

Some men find that their partner is the one with the elevated level of sexual desire. Approximately 10 percent of women experience an *increase* in sexual desire at some point during The Pause. This may be because of *increased* testosterone levels or the end of worry about getting pregnant or no longer having to be concerned about children listening in the next room. You may find your partner's increased desire a major bonus—or you may discover that she is getting warmed up just as you are beginning to cool off.

At this time in life you may be experiencing a change in your own sexuality. You may find it takes longer to get an erection. You may need more direct physical stimulation of your penis to get erect. And you may lose your erection more easily than you have in the past. Your erections may be less firm, your ejaculate less copious, and you may not experience orgasm every time you make love. Some of these changes are due to the slowly decreasing levels of free testosterone that frequently accompany the aging process. Everything slows down as we age, but if we are not prepared, these natural physiological changes can cause anxiety, depression, or feelings of inadequacy that can further interfere with sexual responsiveness.

If your partner is experiencing pain with intercourse or seems less interested in you as a lover, it may be the final straw that causes you to give up on sex altogether ... or at least with her. It may be easier to lay your sexuality to rest than anticipate the possibility of sexual "failure."

At this time of life, fears of losing attractiveness and virility can lead some men to an affair with a younger woman. An affair with a twenty- or thirty-something-year-old can intensify your sexual feelings and responses and be just the elixir to make you feel young again, but this drastic decision can have devastating consequences for any relationship. Needless to say, it is important to ascertain whether your sexual or marital difficulties lie in a midlife crisis or are truly the result of relationship problems with your partner before taking action that can cause irreparable harm.

"I respect and love my wife and we have two wonderful children, but I nearly left her for another woman. There was an excitement yet a depth in this other relationship, more powerful than anything I had ever experienced. I really felt we were soul-mates. I miss her terribly. Of course, I'll never know what would have happened, because I stayed in my marriage. My affair catapulted us into a crisis that forced us to make some major changes. I think we are both happier as a result. And I can't say enough how I appreciate my wife for sticking with it and doing her part so we could get to where we are now."

If you want to maintain your sexual relationship, you probably will have to adapt your lovemaking to the physical changes you are both experiencing. For many couples, this means less intercourse and more touching, self-pleasuring, and oral sex. It means dropping the belief that orgasm must always occur for the lovemaking to be satisfying.

What you get out of sex now may be different from before. For example, in a *Longevity* magazine survey, we found that while intercourse and orgasm ranked highest for men in their younger years, once they entered their forties, pleasing their partner and expressing love became most important.

Closeness, intimacy, and sexual pleasure are available throughout our lives if we keep the nonsexual part of the relationship satisfying and if we maintain our good health.

If marital problems are overwhelming you, see a therapist. Even after twenty-five years of an unsatisfying marriage, many couples are able to start over again once they learn the skills necessary to resolve their problems. Each relationship has its unique difficulties. Just relating to yourself can be problematic enough—when you add a partner with her own needs and ideas, difficulties are multiplied exponentially.

This is not to say that all couples should stay together. Some couples are suited for childrearing, for example, yet find they have little in common once the children move out. However, it is hard to argue with the idea that the best way to grow older is with someone you trust and love, someone with whom you have weathered many of life's inevitable storms. Working together, with support and love, through The Pause until you get to the other side can secure the relationship for a lifetime.

Further Information

Lonnie Barbach, Ph.D., and David L. Geisinger, Ph.D. *Going the Distance: Finding and Keeping Lifelong Love.* New York: Plume, 1993.

Summary of Symptoms and Solutions

Premenstrual syndrome, mood swings, irritability, depression

    Diet—Avoid alcohol, sugar, dairy products, salt

    Exercise—Daily

    Behavior—Relax whenever necessary

      Prepare family members and colleagues

      Undergo psychotherapy when needed

      Don't smoke

    Supplements—Vitamin B-6: 50–300 milligrams per day

      Magnesium: 150–400 milligrams per day

    Homeopathy—Individual remedies

    Acupuncture and Chinese herbs—Individual treatment

    Herbs—Chasteberry (Vitex)

      Skullcap for irritability

      Saint-John's-wort for depression

    Hormones—Estrogen is particularly effective

      Natural progesterone

Fatigue

Exercise—Daily
Homeopathy—Individual remedies
Acupuncture and Chinese herbs—Individual treatment
Herbs—Chasteberry (Vitex)
Hormones—Estrogen (sometimes testosterone)

Sleep disturbance

Diet—Avoid caffeinated and alcoholic beverages
    Avoid large evening meals
    Drink warm milk before bedtime
Exercise—Daily
Behavior—White noise, very hot baths, reading, relaxation exercises
Homeopathy—Individual remedies
Acupuncture and Chinese herbs—Individual treatment
Herbs—Motherwort, passionflower, valerian
Hormones—Estrogen

Mental fuzziness

Behavior—Increase organization, use notes and lists
Homeopathy—Individual remedies
Acupuncture and Chinese herbs—Individual treatment
Herbs—Chasteberry (Vitex)
Hormones—Estrogen is particularly effective

Joint and muscle pain

Behavior—Massage
Exercise—Daily
Homeopathy—Individual remedies
Acupuncture and Chinese herbs—Particularly helpful
Herbs—Burdock, black cohosh, blue cohosh, nettles, cleavers for joint pain
Hormones—Estrogen

Gastric upset, constipation, diarrhea

Homeopathy—Individual remedies are particularly effective

Acupuncture and Chinese herbs—Individual treatment

Herbs—Chamomile tea, peppermint tea, bitter herbs for gastric upset, psyllium husks for constipation

Hormones—Estrogen

Nausea and dizziness

Homeopathy—Individual remedies

Acupuncture and Chinese herbs—Individual treatment

Herbs—Chasteberry (Vitex)

Headaches

Homeopathy—Individual remedies are particularly effective

Acupuncture and Chinese herbs—Individual treatment

Herbs—Chasteberry (Vitex), peppermint oil, feverfew

Hormones—Estrogen

Skin sensitivity

Homeopathy—Individual remedies

Acupuncture and Chinese herbs—Individual treatment

Herbs—Chasteberry (Vitex)

Hormones—Estrogen

Breast tenderness

Supplements—Vitamin E: 100–800 international units per day

Homeopathy—Individual remedies

Acupuncture and Chinese herbs—Individual treatment

Herbs—Chasteberry (Vitex)

Hormones—Progesterone or testosterone

Frequent urination

Homeopathy—Individual remedies

Acupuncture and Chinese herbs—Individual treatment

Herbs—Chasteberry (Vitex)

Hormones—Estrogen—Estrogen cream may be sufficient

Urinary incontinence

Behavior—Kegel exercises, relaxing while voiding

Homeopathy—Individual remedies

Acupuncture and Chinese herbs—Individual treatment

Herbs—Chasteberry (Vitex)

Hormones—Estrogen for urge incontinence

Medical—Surgery

Hot flashes

Supplements—Vitamin E: 600–800 international units per day

Hesperidin: 1,000 milligrams per day

Vitamin C: 500–1,000 milligrams three times per day

Diet—Avoid coffee, chocolate, alcohol, spicy foods, and fruits high in acid

Keep cold liquids nearby

Exercise—Daily

Behavior—Dress in layers, carry a fan, have sex weekly

Homeopathy—Individual remedies

Acupuncture and Chinese herbs—Individual treatment

Herbs—Chasteberry (Vitex), black cohosh, Dong Quai, Siberian ginseng

Hormones—Estrogen is particularly effective (sometimes progesterone or testosterone)

Medical—Clonidine, Aldomet

Heart palpitations
> Homeopathy—Individual remedies
> Acupuncture and Chinese herbs—Individual treatment
> Herbs—Chasteberry (Vitex), black cohosh, Dong Quai
> Hormones—Estrogen
> Behavior—Relaxation

Heavy bleeding
> Acupuncture and Chinese herbs—particularly effective
> Homeopathy—Individual remedies
> Herbs—Chasteberry (Vitex), shepherd's purse, blessed
>   thistle
> Hormones—Progesterone
> Medical—D&C, ablation or laser burning of the uterine
>   lining, hysterectomy

Weight gain
> Exercise—Aerobic, daily
> Diet—Reduce intake of fats
>   Drink lots of water

Hair loss
> Homeopathy—Individual remedies
> Acupuncture and Chinese herbs—Individual treatment
> Herbs—Chasteberry (Vitex)
> Hormones—Estrogen
> Medical—Antitestosterone medication plus Rogain

Increased hair growth
> Behavior—Bleaching, electrolysis
> Hormone—Estrogen or natural progesterone
> Medical—Antitestosterone medication

Skin problems

    Behavior—Quit smoking
      Use sunscreen
    Diet—Drink lots of water
    Homeopathy—Individual remedies
    Acupuncture and Chinese herbs—Individual treatment
    Herbs—Chasteberry (Vitex)
    Hormones—Estrogen for dry skin
      Natural progesterone cream for acne
    Medical—Retin-A or antitestosterone medication for acne

Lack of sexual desire

    Behavior—Psychotherapy when appropriate
    Homeopathy—Individual remedies
    Acupuncture and Chinese herbs—Individual treatment
    Herbs—Chasteberry (Vitex)
    Hormones—Estrogen and/or testosterone

Painful intercourse

    Behavior—Additional lubrication with sex
      Vitamin E or Replens on regular basis
      Masturbation and stretching vagina
      Psychotherapy when appropriate
    Homeopathy—Individual remedies
    Acupuncture and Chinese herbs—Individual treatment
    Herbs—Chasteberry (Vitex)
    Hormones—Estrogen—cream or pills—is particularly effective
      Natural progesterone cream
      Testosterone cream
    Supplements—Zinc: 15 milligrams per day

Heart disease prevention

Exercise—Aerobic, minimum three times per week

Diet—nonfat or low-fat, low-cholesterol, moderate fiber

Hormones—Estrogen

Supplements—Vitamin C: 500–3,000 milligrams per day

Vitamin E: over 100 international units per day

Miscellaneous—Baby aspirin: one per day

Osteoporosis

Exercise—Weight-bearing: three hours per week minimum

Diet—Consume adequate dairy products; increase other foods high in calcium

Drink calcium-fortified juices

Decrease animal flesh significantly

Supplements—Total intake from food plus supplements:

Calcium (elemental): 800 milligrams per day with estrogen

Calcium (elemental): 1,200–1,500 milligrams per day without estrogen

Vitamin D: 400 international units per day

Magnesium: 150–400 milligrams per day

Malic acid, boric acid, manganese, silicon, copper, zinc

Hormones—Estrogen and testosterone

Chapter 1

p. 12   "continued to feel that way": N. E. Avis and S. M. McKinlay, "A longitudinal analysis of women's attitudes toward the menopause: results from the Massachusetts Women's Health Study," *Maturitas*, 13:1 (1991), pp. 65–79.

Chapter 2

p. 15   "they have stiff shoulders": B. M. du Toit, "Aging and Menopause Among Indian South African Women," SUNY Series M Medical Anthropology, State University of New York Press, 1990, p. 9.

p. 15   "no physical complaints at all": Y. Beyene, "Cultural significance and physiological manifestations of menopause: a biocultural analysis," *Culture, Med Psychiatry*, vol. 10 (1986), p. 58.

p. 15   "those of Western women": B. Moore and H. Kombe, "Climacteric symptoms in a Tanzanian community," *Maturitas*, 13:3 (1991), p. 232.

p. 15   "with virtually no discomfort": M. Flint, "The menopause: reward or punishment?" *Psychosomatics*, 16:3 (1975), p. 162; D. M. Barbo, "The physiology of the menopause," *Medical Clinics of North America,* 71:1 (1987), p. 11.

p. 16   "so severe they are incapacitated": M. Flint, "The menopause"; D. M. Barbo, "The physiology of the menopause." Ibid.

p. 25   "unless absolutely necessary": W. B. Cutler, *Hysterectomy: Before and After* (New York: Harper & Row, 1988).

p. 26   "earlier time in their lives": J. B. McKinlay, S. M. McKinlay, and D. Brambilla, "The relative contributions of endocrine changes and social circumstances to depression in mid-aged women," *J Health and Behavior,* 28:4 (1987), p. 347.

Chapter 3

p. 30   "to about age eighty-one": "Vital Statistics of the United States, 1988, life tables," U.S. Dept. of Health and Human Services Pub. No. (PHS) 91-1104, vol. 11, section 6.

p. 31   "who have gone through it": M. S. Hunter, "Emotional well-being, sexual behavior and hormone replacement therapy," *Maturitas,* 12:3 (1990), p. 305.

p. 31   "many others in life": A. A. Quinn, "A theoretical model of the perimenopausal process," *J Nurse-Midwifery,* 36:1 (1991), p. 28.

p. 31   "about their mental health": N. Datan, "Aging into transitions: cross-cultural perspectives on women at midlife," in R. Formanek (ed.), *The Meanings of Menopause: Historical, Medical and Clinical Perspectives* (Hillsdale, NJ: Analytic Press, 1990), p. 129.

p. 32   "at work and home": D. J. Cooke, "A psychological study of the climacteric," in A. Brooke and L. Wallace (eds.), *Psychology and Gynaecological Problems* (London: Tavistock Publications, 1984).

p. 33   "a number of studies": C. A. Mose, "Menopausal mood disorders," *Comprehensive Therapy,* 15:3 (1989), p. 24; and W. B. Cutler and C.-R. García, *Love Cycles: The Science of Intimacy* (New York: Villard Books, 1991).

p. 36   "the premenopausal years": M. Hunter, R. Battersby, and M. Whitehead, "Relationships between psychological symptoms, somatic complaints and menopausal status," *Maturitas,* 8 (1986), pp. 217–28.

p. 37   "one of significant mourning": M. Lock, "Ambiguities of aging: Japanese experience and perceptions of meno-pause," *Culture, Med Psychiatry,* vol. 10 (1986), p. 23.

p. 38   "Cambridge, Massachusetts": J. B. McKinlay, S. M. McKinlay, and D. Brambilla, "The relative contribu-tions of endocrine changes and social circumstances to depression in mid-aged women," *J Health and Behavior,* 28:4 (1987), p. 353.

p. 38   "evidenced . . . greater depression": D. Kritz-Silverstein, D. Wingard, E. Barrett-Connor, D. Morton, "Hysterec-tomy, oophorectomy and depression in older women," presented at the Fourth Annual Meeting of the North American Menopause Society, San Diego, California, Sept. 2–4, 1993.

p. 39   "estrogen levels are lowest": E. S. Abramowitz, A. H. Bakerk, and S. F. Fleischer, "Onset of depressive psychi-atric crisis and the menstrual cycle," *American Journal of Psychiatry,* vol. 139 (1982), pp. 475–78.

p. 39   "suicidal thoughts went down": P. Sarrel: "Ovarian hor-mones and the circulation, quiz the panel," presented at the Third Annual Meeting of the North American Menopause Society, Case Western Reserve University, Cleveland, Ohio, Sept. 17–20, 1992.

p. 43   "can be a real blessing": E. L. Klaiber, D. M. Broverman, W. Vogel, and Y. Kobayashi, "Estrogen therapy for severe persistent depressions in women," *Arch General Psych,* 36:5 (1978), p. 550; H. Hafner, S. Behrens, J. DeVry, and W. F. Gattaz, "An animal model for the effects of estradiol on dopamine-mediated behavior: implications for sex differences in schizophre-nia," *Psychiatry Research,* 38:2 (1991), pp. 125–34.

p. 44   "enhanced mood": M. Aylward, "Plasma tryptophan levels in perimenopausal patients," in S. Campbell (ed.), *The Management of the Menopause and Post-Menopausal Years* (Baltimore: University Park Press, 1976).

p. 44   "serious depression": B. Sherwin, "Sex hormones and mood: clinical research," presented at the Fourth An-nual meeting of the North American Menopause Soci-ety, San Diego, California, Sept. 2–4, 1993.

p. 44   "more effective than Premarin": E. L. Vliet and L. Lewis, "Differential response in CNS menopausal symptoms between 17-beta-estradiol and conjugated es-trogens," presented at the Fourth Annual Meeting of the North American Menopause Society, San Diego, California, Sept. 2–4, 1993.

p. 46   "emotional symptoms of PMS": H. Doll, S. Brown, A. Thurston and M. Vessey, "Pyridoxine (vitamin B6) and the premenstrual syndrome: a randomized crossover trial," *Journal of the Royal College of General Practitioners,* 326:39 (1989), pp. 364–68.

p. 46   "(Optivite, Rejuvex, Pro-Woman, and de Buren's . . .": Optivite is carried in many pharmacies. Rejuvex can be found in health food stores. Pro-Woman may be mail-ordered (800-KICK-PMS). De Buren's Optimum International may also be mail-ordered (800-543-3831).

p. 46   "problems in high doses": J. E. Brody, "Natural remedies can help menopausal women," *San Diego Union-Tribune,* May 27, 1992, p. E-2; P. J. Fahey, J. M. Boltri, and J. S. Monk, "Key issues in nutrition: supplementation through adulthood and old age," *Postgraduate Med,* 81:6 (1987), pp. 123–28.

p. 47   "control PMS symptoms": G. S. Goei and G. E. Abraham, "Effect of a nutritional supplement, Optivite, on symptoms of premenstrual tension," *J Reproductive Med,* 28:8 (1983), p. 527.

p. 47   "and nervous tension": G. E. Abraham, "Nutritional factors in the etiology of the premenstrual tension syndromes," *J Reproductive Med,* 28:7 (1983), pp. 451–52.

p. 48   "chronic magnesium deficiency": Fahey, Boltri, and Monk, p. 452.

p. 48   "by depleting potassium": D. Ullman, *Discovering Homeopathy: Medicine for the 21st Century* (Berkeley, CA: North Atlantic Books, 1991), p. 109.

p. 49   "be depressed during it": M. S. Hunter, "Somatic experience of the menopause: a prospective study," *Psychosom Med,* 52:3, p. 365.

p. 49   "less negative mood": A. Collins and B. Landgren, "Reproductive health, estrogen use and experience of symptoms in perimenopausal women," presented at the Fourth Annual Meeting of the North American Menopause Society, San Diego, California, Sept. 2–4, 1993.

Chapter 4

p. 55   "companions of The Pause": M. Mauri, Ph.D., "Sleep and the reproductive cycle: a review," *Health Care for Women Int'l,* 11:4 (1990), p. 416.

p. 55   "of home and job": Statistical Abstract of the United States, 1992, U.S. Bureau of the Census, 112th Edition.

p. 58   "sleep complaints": J. M. Fry, "Sleep disorders," *Medical Clinics of North America*, 71:1 (1987), p. 100.

p. 59   "estrogen levels are lowest": Mauri, "Sleep and the reproductive cycle," p. 410.

p. 59   "reported by PMS sufferers": Ibid., p. 412.

p. 61   "the early 1960s": E. Jacobson, *You Must Relax* (New York: McGraw-Hill, 1962).

p. 61   "The Relaxation Response": H. Benson, *The Relaxation Response* (New York: Avon Books, 1976).

p. 62   "frequency of awakenings": J. M. Fry, "Sleep disorders," *Medical Clinics of North America*, 71:1 (1987), p. 105.

p. 62   "to feel rested and well": Ibid.

p. 62   "associated with sleep": S. Mondini, M. Zucconi, F. Cirigonotta et al., "Snoring as a risk factor for cardiac and circulatory problems: an epidemiological study," in C. Guilleminault and E. Lugaresi (eds.), *Sleep/Wake Disorders: Natural History, Epidemiology, and Long-Term Evolution* (New York: Raven Press, 1983); J. Thomson, "Double-blind study on the effect of estrogen on sleep, anxiety and depression in perimenopausal women: preliminary results," *Royal Soc Med Proc*, vol. 69 (1976), pp. 829–30; J. Thomson and I. Oswald, "Effects of estrogen on the sleep, mood and anxiety of menopausal women," *Br Med J*, 2:6098 (1977), pp. 1317–19.

p. 65   "measures of cognitive functioning": B. B. Sherwin, "Estrogen and memory in postmenopausal women," presented at Third Annual Meeting, North American Menopause Society, Case Western Reserve University, Cleveland, Ohio, Sept. 17–20, 1992.

p. 65   "93 percent reduction": S. J. Birge, "The role of estrogens in falls, fractures and dementia," presented at the Fourth Annual Meeting of the North American Menopause Society, San Diego, California, Sept. 2–4, 1993.

p. 66   "estrogen withdrawal symptoms": S. Ballinger, D. Cobbin, J. Krivanek, and D. Saunders, "Life stresses and depression in the menopause," *Maturitas*, 1 (1979), pp. 191–99; and S. Ballinger, "The role of psychosocial stress in menopausal symptoms," in L. Carenza and L. Zichella (eds.), *Emotions and Reproduction*, vol. 20B, Proceedings of the Serono Symposia (London: Academic Press, 1979), pp. 1239–45.

p. 66   "children still at home": S. B. Phillips, "Reflections of
           self and other: men's views of menopausal women," in
           R. Formanek (ed.), *The Meanings of Menopause: Historical,
           Medical and Clinical Perspectives* (Hillsdale, NJ: Analytic
           Press, 1990), p. 288.

p. 67   "rather than personal satisfaction": M. S. Hunter,
           "Emotional well-being, sexual behavior and hormone
           replacement therapy," *Maturitas*, 12:3 (1990), p. 304.

p. 67   "transition through menopause": J. G. Greene, "Psy-
           chosocial influences and life events at the time of the
           menopause," in R. Formanek (ed.), *The Meanings of
           Menopause*, pp. 86, 88; Y. Beyene, "Cultural significance
           and physiological manifestations of menopause: a
           biocultural analysis," *Culture, Med Psychiatry*, vol. 10
           (1986), p. 48; Hunter, "Emotional well-being"; P. A.
           van Keep and J. M. Kellerhals, "The impact of socio-
           cultural factors on symptom formation: some results of
           a study on aging women in Switzerland," *Psychother
           Psychosom*, vol. 23 (1–6) (1974), pp. 251–63.

p. 67   "fewer somatic symptoms": Greene, "Psychosocial influ-
           ences," p. 84.

p. 67   "through this period": L. Dennerstain, "Depression in
           the menopause," *Obstetrics and Gynecology Clinics of North
           America*, 14:1 (1987), p. 44.

p. 67   *"Healing Yourself"*: M. L. Rossman, *Healing Yourself* (New
           York: Pocket Books, 1987).

p. 68   "B complex twice a day": J. Crerand, "Home remedy:
           insomnia," *Natural Health*, Mar./Apr. 1992, p. 100.

p. 68   "can also be helpful": P. J. Fahey, J. M. Boltri, and J. S.
           Monk, "Key issues in nutrition: supplementation
           through adulthood and old age," *Postgraduate Med*, 81:6
           (1987), p. 128.

Chapter 5

p. 71   "joint and bone pain": F. E. Okonofua, A. Lawal, and
           J. K. Bamgbose, "Features of menopause and meno-
           pausal age in Nigerian women," *Int'l J Gynecol Obstet*,
           31:4 (1990), p. 343.

p. 71   "stiff or sore shoulders": M. Lock, P. Kaufert, and P. Gil-
           bert, "Cultural construction of the menopausal syndrome:
           the Japanese case," *Maturitas*, 10:4 (1988), p. 324.

p. 71   "frozen shoulders": H. P. Kopell, W. A. Thompson,

"Pain and the frozen shoulder," *Surg Gynecol Obstet,* vol. 109 (1959), pp. 92–96.

p. 72   "cause stomach upset": T. Sakaguchi, M. Yamazaki, S. Itoh, N. Okamura, and T. Banko, "Gastric acid secretion controlled by oestrogen in women," *J Int'l Med Res,* 19:5 (1991), pp. 384–88.

p. 73   "going through The Pause": C. A. Mose, "Menopausal mood disorders," *Comprehensive Therapy,* 15:3 (1989), p. 24.

p. 79   "to have the problem": P. Rousseau and A. Fuentevilla-Clifton, "Urinary incontinence in the aged, Part 1: patient evaluation," *Geriatrics,* 47:6 (1992), p. 22.

p. 79   "control urinary incontinence": A. H. Kegel, "Progressive resistance exercise in the functional restoration of the perineal muscles," *Am J Obstet Gynecol,* vol. 56 (1948), p. 238.

p. 80   "of female patients": P. Rousseau and A. Fuentevilla-Clifton, "Urinary incontinence in the aged, Part 2: management strategies," *Geriatrics,* 47:6 (1992), pp. 37–39; J. Baigis-Smith, D. A. Jakovac Smith, M. Rose, and D. Kaschak Newman, "Managing urinary incontinence in community-residing elderly persons," *Gerontologist,* 29:2 (1989), pp. 229–33.

p. 81   "the PC muscle": K. L. Burgio, J. C. Robinson, and B. T. Engel, "The role of biofeedback in Kegel exercise training for stress urinary incontinence," *Am J Obstet Gynecol,* 154:1 (1986), p. 60.

p. 82   "proper acid balance": M. M. Gelfand and E. Wendman, "An evaluation of a bioadhesive vaginal moisturizing gel in women with breast cancer," presented at the Second Annual Meeting of the North American Menopause Society, Montreal, Canada, Sept. 25–28, 1991.

p. 83   "during The Pause": C. A. Mose, "Menopausal mood disorders," *Comprehensive Therapy,* 15:3 (1989), p. 24.

p. 83   "will seek treatment": Ibid., p. 23.

p. 87   "at least for a while": D. C. Harper, "Perimenopause and Aging," in R. Lichtman and S. Papera (eds.), *Gynecology: Well-Woman Care* (Norwalk, CT: Appleton & Lange, 1990), p. 408.

p. 88   "sporadically for decades": D. M. Barbo, "The physiology of the menopause," *Medical Clinics of North America,* 71:1 (1987), p. 15.

p. 88   "Japanese word for it": M. Lock, "Ambiguities of aging:

Japanese experience and perceptions of menopause," *Culture, Med Psychiatry,* vol. 10 (1986), p. 37.

p. 88   "report having hot flashes": F. E. Okonofua, A. Lawal, and J. K. Bamgbose, "Features of menopause and menopausal age in Nigerian women," *Int'l J Gynecol Obstet,* 31:4 (1990), p. 344.

p. 88   "Western-acculturated city-dwellers": M. Fling and R. S. Samil, "Cultural and subcultural meanings of the menopause," *New York Academy of Sciences,* vol. 592 (1990), p. 143.

p. 89   "frequency of hot flashes": L. Swartzman, R. Edelberg, and E. Kemmann, "Impact of stress on objectively recorded menopausal hot flushes and on flush report bias," *Health Psychology,* 9:5 (1990), pp. 529–45.

p. 89   "their hot flashes": J. P. Wallace, S. Lovell, C. Talano, M. L. Webb, and J. L. Hodgson, "Changes in menstrual function, climacteric syndrome, and serum concentrations of sex hormones in pre- and post-menopausal women following a moderate intensity conditioning program," *Med Sci in Sports & Exercise,* vol. 14 (1982), p. 154.

p. 89   "recent biofeedback study": R. R. Freedman and S. Woodward, "Behavioral treatment of menopausal hot flushes: Evaluation by ambulatory monitoring," *Am J Obstet Gynecol,* 167:2 (1992), pp. 436–39.

p. 91   "some are purse size": Brookstone retail stores carry them.

p. 92   "less intense hot flashes": N. McCoy, W. Cutler, and J. M. Davidson, "Relationships among sexual behavior, hot flashes and hormone levels in peri-menopausal women," *Arch Sex Beh,* vol. 14 (1985), pp. 385–94.

p. 92   "1,000 milligrams a day is taken": J. Reichenberg-Ullman, "Menopause naturally," *Natural Health,* Mar./Apr. (1992), p. 78.

p. 93   "electro-stimulated acupuncture": A. M. Hammar, R. Lindgren, Y. Wyon, and T. Lundberg, "Does acupuncture influence the frequency of post menopausal hot flushes?" presented at the Second Annual Meeting of the North American Menopause Society, Montreal, Canada, Sept. 25–28, 1991.

p. 99   "within their lifetime": A. Treloar, "Menstrual cyclicity and the pre-menopause," *Maturitas,* 3 (1981), pp. 249–64; B. C. Richards, "Hysterectomy: from women

to women," *Am J Obstet Gynecol,* vol. 131 (1~~~~
446–49.

p. 99   "other European countries": W. B. Cutler, *Hysterectomy: Before and After* (New York: Harper & Row, 1990), p. 2.

p. 99   "under the knife": For more information read Cutler, *Hysterectomy: Before and After.* Ibid.

p. 100   "experience of orgasm": W. B. Cutler, "The behavioral endocrinology of sexuality as women age," presented at the Second Annual Meeting of the North American Menopause Society, Montreal, Canada, Sept. 25–28, 1991.

p. 100   "their ovaries removed": R. G. Dicker, M. J. Scally, J. R. Greenspan, P. M. Layde, and J. M. Maze, "Hysterectomy among women of reproductive age," *JAMA,* vol. 243 (1982), pp. 323–27.

p. 100   "iron tablet supplements": Reichenberg-Ullman, "Menopause naturally," *Natural Health* (Mar./Apr. 1992), p. 80.

p. 100   "when their periods end": S. M. McKinlay and M. Jefferys, "The menopausal syndrome," *Br J Prev Soc Med,* 28:2 (1974), pp. 108–15; M. McKinlay and J. B. McKinlay, "Health status and health care utilization by menopausal women," in M. Notelovitz and P. A. Van Keep (eds.), *The Climacteric in Perspective: Proceedings of the fourth international congress on the menopause* (Lancaster, England: MTP Press Ltd, 1986); K. Garde and I. Lunde, "Female sexual behavior. A study in a random sample of 40-year-old women," *Maturitas,* 2 (1980), pp. 225–40.

p. 101   "in different generations": S. M. McKinlay and M. Jefferys, "The menopausal syndrome," *Br J Prev Soc Med,* 28 (1974), pp. 108–15.

p. 101   "among different cultures": M. Lock, "Ambiguities of aging: Japanese experience and perceptions of menopause," *Culture Med Psychiatry,* vol. 10 (1986), pp. 23–46.

Chapter 6

p. 105   "had gained weight": J. Wurtman, J. Cobb, J. McDermott, and R. Gleason, "Menopause and weight gain among normal and obese women," presented at the Third Annual Meeting of the North American Menopause Society, Case Western Reserve University, Cleveland, Ohio, Sept. 17–20, 1992.

p. 105   "controlling weight": C. S. Berkun, "In behalf of

women over 40: Understanding the importance of the menopause," *Social Work*, Sept./Oct. 1986, p. 380.

pp. 106   "throughout adult life": M. R. Sutnick, "Nutrition: calcium, cholesterol and calories," *Medical Clinics of North America*, 71:1 (1987), p. 130.

p. 106   "more than men": J. Wurtman et al., "Menopause and weight gain among normal and obese women."

p. 107   "progesterone are decreasing": W. B. Cutler and C.-R. García, *Love Cycles: The Science of Intimacy* (New York: Villard Books, 1991), p. 70.

p. 109   "who have heart attacks": J. Haarbo, U. Marslew, A. Gotfredsen, and C. Christiansen, "Postmenopausal hormone replacement therapy prevents central distribution of body fat after menopause," *Metabolism*, 40:12 (1991), pp. 1323–26.

p. 109   "lowest exercise levels": R. R. Wing, K. A. Matthews, L. H. Kuller, E. N. Meilahn, and P. L. Plantings, "Weight gain at the time of menopause," *Arch Intern Med*, 151:1 (1991), p. 101.

p. 113   "hide or eliminate it": A small appliance called Finally Free, manufactured by Selvac Corporation, can be used to eliminate increased facial and body hair.

p. 113   "hair growth for 93 percent": A. Ostrzenski, "Treatment of androgenetic alopecia in postmenopausal women," presented at the Third Annual Meeting of the North American Menopause Society, Case Western Reserve University, Cleveland, Ohio, Sept. 17–20, 1992.

p. 115   "smoking is antiestrogenic": D. L. Cassidente, A. G. Vijod, M. A. Vijod, F. Z. Stoncgyk, and R. A. Lobo, "Short term effects of smoking on the pharmacokinetic profiles of micronized estradiol in postmenopausal women," *Am J Obstet Gynecol*, vol. 163 (1990), pp. 1953–60.

p. 116   "ever in her career": A. Kahn, "A guide for women and the men who love them," *San Francisco Chronicle*, Apr. 17, 1992, p. D-3-5.

p. 117   "will be over fifty": "Statistical abstracts of the United States 1991," U.S. Department of Commerce, Economics and Statistics Administration, Bureau of the Census.

Chapter 7

p. 119   "80 percent of us": M. S. Hunter, R. Battersby, and M. Whitehead, "Relationships between psychological symptoms, somatic complaints and menopausal status,"

Maturitas, 8 (1986), pp. 217–28; M. S. Hunter, "Psychological and somatic experience of the menopause: A prospective study," *Psychosom Med,* vol. 52 (1990), pp. 357–67.

p. 119   "safe and effective solutions": P. M. Sarrel, "Sexuality and menopause," *Obstet Gynecol,* 75:4 (1990), p. 29S.

p. 121   "their younger years": P. M. Sarrel, "Sexuality and menopause"; R. K. McCraw, "Psychosexual changes associated with the perimenopausal period," *J Nurse-Midwifery,* 36:1 (1991), p. 18.

p. 124   "comfort during intercourse": M. M. Gelfand and E. Wendman, "An evaluation of a bioadhesive vaginal moisturizing gel in women with breast cancer," presented at the Second Annual Meeting of the North American Menopause Society, Montreal, Canada, Sept. 25–28, 1991.

p. 124   "rich in zinc": D. C. Harper, "Perimenopause and aging," in R. Lichtman and S. Papera (eds.), *Gynecology: Well-Woman Care* (Norwalk, CT: Appleton & Lange, 1990).

p. 125   "from sexual discomfort": L. Mettler and P. G. Olsen, "Long-term treatment of atrophic vaginitis with low-dose oestradiol vaginal tablets," *Maturitas,* 14 (1991), pp. 23–31.

p. 126   "six weeks of supplementation": G. Wilcox, M. L. Wahlqvist, H. G. Burger, G. Medley, "Oestrogenic effects of plant foods in postmenopausal women," *Br Med J,* 301 (1990), pp. 905–6.

p. 128   "insufficient testosterone": H. S. Kaplan, "A neglected issue: The sexual side effects of current treatments for breast cancer," *J Sex & Marital Therapy,* 18:1 (1992), p. 8.

p. 128   "are not significant": M. S. Hunter, "Emotional well-being, sexual behavior and hormone replacement therapy," *Maturitas,* 12:3 (1990), p. 303.

p. 128   "diminish sexual enjoyment": Ibid.

p. 130   "purchased by mail": Good Vibrations, 1210 Valencia St., San Francisco, CA 94110, (415) 974-8990, sells books and sexual products for women and couples.

p. 131   "keeps the vagina healthy": S. Leiblum, G. Bachmann, E. Kemmann, D. Colburn, and L. Swartzman, "Vaginal atrophy in the postmenopausal woman: the importance of sexual activity and hormones," *JAMA,* vol. 249 (1983), pp. 2195–98.

p. 132   "at least 35 percent": G. A. Bachmann, "Sexual problems during the menopause," presented at the Menopausal Syndrome Symposium, Scottsdale, AZ, Jan. 27, 1990.

p. 132   "for others, permanent": S. E. Ballinger and E. C. Howe, "Sexual problems in a menopause clinic: Some ideas on aetiology and incidence," paper presented at the Third International Congress on the Menopause, Ostend, Belgium, 1981; W. B. Cutler and C.-R. García, *Menopause: A Guide for Women and the Men Who Love Them* (New York: W. W. Norton, 1992).

p. 133   "for three to six months": P. M. Sarrel, "Sex and Menopause," presented at the Second Annual Meeting of the North American Menopause Society, Montreal, Canada, Sept. 25–28, 1991.

p. 134   "prior to the actual menopause": Chris Longcope, M.D., personal communication.

p. 137   "and blood lipid levels": G. G. Burger, J. Hailes, M. Menelaus, J. Nelson, B. Hudson, and N. Balazs, "The management of persistent menopausal symptoms with oestradiol-testosterone implants: clinical, lipid and hormonal results," *Maturitas*, 6 (1984), pp. 351–58; B. B. Sherwin, M. M. Gelfand, R. Schucher and J. Gabor, "Postmenopausal estrogen and androgen replacement and lipoprotein lipid concentrations," *Am J Obstet Gynec*, 156:2 (1987), pp. 414–19; R. Greenblatt, "Androgens in clinical practice: Part I—In the female," *Today's Therapeutic Trends*, 4:1 (1986), pp. 31–47.

p. 139   "or after The Pause": A. Koster, "Change of life anticipations, attitudes and experiences among middle-aged Danish women," *Health Care for Women Int'l*, 12:1 (1991), p. 8.

p. 140   "fifties than women": G. T. Bungay, M. P. Vessay, and C. K. McPherson, "Study of symptoms in middle life with special reference to the menopause," *Br Med J*, vol. 2 (1980), pp. 181–83.

p. 140   "their sexual relationship": E. Pfeiffer, A. Verwoerdt, and G. C. Davis, "Sexual behavior in middle life," *Am J Psychiatry*, vol. 128 (1972), pp. 1262–67.

p. 143   "the most important part": B. Starr and M. Weiner, *The Starr-Weiner Report on Sex and Sexuality in the Mature Years* (New York: McGraw-Hill, 1981), p. 254.

p. 144   "less severe hot flashes": W. B. Cutler and C.-R. García, *Love Cycles: The Science of Intimacy* (New York: Villard Books, 1991), p. 39.

p. 144   "noticed a decrease": Koster, "Change of life anticipations," pp. 8–9.

Chapter 8

p. 147   "thinking, however, has changed": M. L'Hermite, "Risks of estrogens and progestogens," *Maturitas*, 12 (1990), pp. 215–46.

p. 156   *"not* taking hormone replacement": M. I. Whitehead, "Prevention of endometrial abnormalities," *Acta Obstet Gynaecol Scand*, supp. vol. 134 (1986), pp. 81–91; B. E. Ettinger, "Hormone replacement therapy and coronary heart disease," *Obstetrics and Gynecology Clinics of North America*, 17:4 (1990), p. 749.

p. 156   "natural progesterone cream": Natural Pro-Gest cream is available through Professional and Technical Services, Inc., Portland, OR 97232.

p. 157   "a lessened libido": L. Dennerstein, G. D. Burrows, G. J. Hyman et al., "Hormone therapy and affect," *Maturitas*, 1 (1979), pp. 247–59; and S. Hammarback, T. Backstrom, J. Holst, et al., "Cyclical mood changes as in the premenstrual syndrome during sequential estrogen-progestogen postmenopausal replacement therapy," *Acta Obstet Gynaecol Scand*, vol. 64 (1985), pp. 393–97.

p. 159   "have periods thereafter": A. Birkenfeld and N. G. Kase, "Menopause medicine: Current treatment options and trends," *Comprehensive Therapy*, 17:7 (1991), p. 42.

p. 161   "monogamous sexual relationships": R. A. Kronmal, C. W. Whitney and S. D. Mumford, "The intrauterine device and pelvic inflammatory disease: the women's health study reanalyzed," *J. Clin Epidemiol*, 4:2 (1991), pp. 109–22.

p. 161   "progesterone is taken orally": J. T. Hargrove, S. C. Sharp, E. Eisenberg and K. G. Osteen, "Endometrial evaluation by transvaginal ultrasonography after 5 years of menopausal hormone replacement therapy with continuous estradiol and progesterone," presented at the Fourth Annual Meeting of the North American Menopause Society, San Diego, California, Sept. 2–4, 1993.

p. 161   "on cholesterol levels": E. Darj, S. Nilsson, O. Axelsson, and D. Hellberg, "Clinical and endometrial effects of oestradiol and progesterone in post-menopausal women," *Maturitas*, 13 (1991), pp. 109–15; J. T. Hargrove, W. S. Maxson, A. C. Wentz, and L. S. Burnett, "Menopausal hormone replacement therapy with

continuous daily oral micronized estradiol and progesterone," *Obstet Gynecol,* vol. 23 (1989), p. 606.

p. 161   "the synthetic progestins": Natural micronized progesterone can be obtained through Madison Pharmaceutical Co., 1-800-558-7046.

p. 162   "and hot flashes": R. Sitruk-Ware, C. Bricaire, B.
DeLignieres, H. Yaneva, and P. Mauvais-Jarvis, "Oral
micronized progesterone," *Contraception,* 36:4 (1987), p.
395.

p. 165   " 'may work equally well' ": J. F. Kemp, J. A. Fryer,
and R. J. Baber, "An alternative regimen of hormone
replacement therapy to improve patient compliance,"
Australia New Zealand J Obstet Gynecol, vol. 29 (1989), pp.
66–69; B. Ettinger, J. Selby, and J. T. Citron, "Hormone replacement therapy using daily Premarin with
medroxy progesterone added every 3 months," presented at the Second Annual Meeting of the North
American Menopause Society, Montreal, Canada, Sept.
25–28, 1991.

p. 169   "progestins are added": M. Sillero-Arenas, M. Delgado-
Rodriguez, R. Rodrigues-Canteras, A. Bueno-
Cavanillas, and R. Galvez-Vargas, "Menopausal
hormone replacement therapy and breast cancer: a
meta-analysis," *Obstet Gynecol,* 79:2 (1992), p. 292.

p. 169   *"Understanding Breast Cancer":* P. Kelly, *Understanding Breast
Cancer* (Philadelphia: Temple University Press, 1992).

p. 170   "developing breast cancer": B. Zumoff, "Hormonal
profiles in women with breast cancer," *Anticancer Research,* vol. 8 (1988), pp. 627–36.

p. 170   "after age thirty": Birkenfeld and Kase, "Menopause
medicine: current treatment options and trends," *Comprehensive Therapy,* 17:7 (1991), p. 40; American Cancer
Society, "Cancer Facts and Figures—1992."

p. 171   "relative with the disease": Kelly, *Understanding Breast
Cancer,* p. 103; D. E. Anderson and M. D. Badzioch,
"Risk of familial breast cancer," *Cancer,* vol. 56 (1985),
pp. 383–87.

p. 171   "increase the risk": Birkenfeld and Kase, "Menopause
medicine"; American Cancer Society, "Cancer Facts
and Figures—1992."

p. 172   "with its development": M. J. Stampfer, S. D. Bechtel,
and O. J. Hunter, "Fat, alcohol, selenium and breast

cancer risk," *Contemporary Ob/GYN*, vol. 20 (1992), pp. 42–47.

p. 172   "than any other": R. A. Hiatt, A. Klatsky, and M. A. Armstrong, "Alcohol and breast cancer," *Preventive Medicine*, 17:6 (1988), p. 683.

p. 173   "against breast cancer": D. P. Rose, "Dietary fiber, phytoestrogens, and breast cancer," *Nutrition*, 8:1 (1992), pp. 47–51.

p. 174   "did not later become pregnant": P. J. DiSaia, "Hormone-replacement therapy in patients with breast cancer," *Cancer Supplement*, 71:4 (1993), pp. 1490–1500.

p. 174   "women not on HRT": P. A. Wingo, P. M. Layde, N. C. Lee, G. Rubin, and H. W. Ory, "The risk of breast cancer in postmenopausal women who have used estrogen replacement therapy," *JAMA* 257:2 (1987), pp. 209–15; W. D. Dupont and D. L. Page, "Menopausal estrogen replacement therapy and breast cancer," *Arch Intern Med*, vol. 151 (1991), pp. 67–72.

p. 174   "a high daily dose of progestin": J. A. Eden, B. G. Wren, and S. Nand, "A study of the effect of hormone-replacement therapy on all-cause mortality and recurrence rate in women with breast carcinoma," presented at the Fourth Annual Meeting of the North American Menopause Society, San Diego, California, Sept. 2–4, 1993.

p. 175   "Megace": Edward Lichten, M.D., personal communication.

Chapter 9

p. 181   "their patients to homeopaths": D. Ullman, *Discovering Homeopathy: Medicine for the 21st Century* (Berkeley, CA: North Atlantic Books, 1991), p. xxi; Bouchayer, "Alternative medicines: a general approach to the French situation," *Complementary Medical Research*, vol. 4 (1990), pp. 4–8; R. Wharton and G. Lewith, "Complementary Medicine and the General Practitioner," *Br Med J*, vol. 292 (1986), pp. 1498–1500.

p. 182   *"Guide to Homeopathic Medicines":* S. Cummings and D. Ullman, *Everybody's Guide to Homeopathic Medicines* (Los Angeles, CA: Jeremy P. Tarcher, Inc., 1984).

p. 183   *"British Medical Journal":* J. Kleijnen, P. Knipschild, and G. ter Riet, "Clinical trials of homeopathy," *Br Med J*, vol. 302 (1991), pp. 316–23.

p. 188   "Female Glandular": Female Glandular is made by
          Dolisos, 3014 Rigel Ave., Las Vegas, NV 89102.

p. 191   *"Guide to Chinese Medicine"*: H. Beinfield and E.
          Korngold, *Between Heaven and Earth: A Guide to Chinese
          Medicine* (New York: Ballantine Books, 1991).

p. 196   "the hormones needed": S. S. Weed, *Menopausal Years*
          (Woodstock, NY: Ash Tree Publishing, 1992), p. 43.

p. 196   "Japanese diet is so high": H. Adlercreutz, E.
          Hamalainen, S. Gorbach, and B. Goldin, "Dietary
          phyto-estrogens and the menopause in Japan," *Lancet*,
          vol. 339 (1992), p. 1233.

Chapter 10

p. 202   "dying of cardiovascular disease": J. D. Cohen, "Car-
          diovascular disease: The case for prevention," presented
          at the Third Annual Meeting of the North American
          Menopause Society, Case Western Reserve University,
          Cleveland, Ohio, Sept. 17–20, 1992, p. 52.

p. 202   "disease than men": J. Sachs, *What Women Should Know
          About Menopause* (New York: Dell, 1991), p. 58.

p. 202   "all heart attacks": Cohen, "Cardiovascular disease," p.
          52.

p. 202   "coronary vascular disease as well": B. Ettinger, "Hor-
          mone replacement therapy and coronary heart disease,"
          Obstetrics and Gynecology Clinics of North America, 17:4
          (1990), p. 746.

p. 203   "approximately 50 percent": E. R. Eichner, "Clearing
          the confusion about cholesterol," *Your Patient and Fitness*,
          4:3 (1990), p. 16; Ettinger, "Hormone replacement
          therapy and coronary heart disease."

p. 203   "with estrogen therapy": M. J. Stampfer, W. C. Willett,
          G. A. Colditz et al., "Postmenopausal estrogen therapy
          and cardiovascular disease," *N Eng J Med*, vol. 325
          (1991), pp. 756–62.

p. 203   "after taking it by mouth": J. Jensen et al., "Long-term
          effects of percutaneous estrogens and oral progesterone
          on serum lipoproteins in postmenopausal women," *Am
          J Obstet Gynecol*, 156:1 (1987), pp. 66–71.

p. 204   "if she became fit": S. N. Blair, H. W. Kohl III, R. S.
          Paffenbarger, D. G. Clark, K. Cooper, and L. W. Gib-
          bons, "Physical fitness and all-cause mortality: A pro-
          spective study of healthy men and women," *JAMA*,
          262:17 (1989), p. 2400.

p. 205   " 'one's quality of life' ": B. L. Drinkwater, "Physical activity and the aging woman," presented at the Third Annual Meeting of the North American Menopause Society, Case Western Reserve University, Cleveland, Ohio, Sept. 17–20, 1992, p. 66.

p. 205   "help from exercise": Blair et al., "Physical fitness and all-cause mortality," pp. 2395–2401.

p. 206   "LDL cholesterol levels": Eichner, "Clearing the confusion about cholesterol," p. 15.

p. 206   "by 10 to 15 percent": Ibid., p. 16.

p. 208   "more than two years": M. J. Stampfer et al.; "Vitamin E consumption and the risk of coronary disease in women," *N Eng J Med*, 338:20 (1993), pp. 1444–49.

p. 211   "of fracture by 50 percent": B. Ettinger, "A practical guide to preventing osteoporosis," *Western J Med*, vol. 149 (1988), p. 692.

p. 212   "milligrams of calcium": B. Ettinger, H. K. Genant, and C. E. Cann, "Postmenopausal bone loss is prevented by treatment with low-dosage estrogen with calcium," *Ann Intern Med*, vol. 106 (1987), p. 44.

p. 213   "increases bone mass": J. Reichenberg-Ullman, "Menopause naturally," *Natural Health*, Mar./Apr. 1992, p. 79.

p. 213   "lost 3.3 percent": E. L. Smith, W. Reddan, and P. E. Smith, "Physical activity and calcium modalities for bone mineral increase in aged women," *Med Sci in Sports & Exercise*, vol. 13 (1981), pp. 60–64.

p. 213   "will be lost": J. Aloia, "Exercise and skeletal health," *J Am Geriatr Soc*, vol. 29 (1981), pp. 104–7; and Smith, "Physical activity and calcium modalities for bone mineral increase in aged women."

p. 213   "less rapidly over time": W. S. Pollitzer and J. J. B. Anderson, "Ethnic and genetic differences in bone mass: a review with a hereditary vs. environmental perspective," *Am J Clin Nutr*, 50:6 (1989), pp. 1244–59.

p. 213   "that of white females": Ibid., p. 1245.

p. 213   "three times as frequently": G. E. Lewinnek, J. Kelsey, A. A. White III, and N. J. Kreiger, "The significance and a comparative analysis of the epidemiology of hip fractures," *Clinical Orthopaedics and Related Research*, no. 152 (1980).

p. 214   "smoking": M. Hernandez-Avila, G. A. Colditz, M. J. Stampfer, B. Rosner, F. E. Speizer, and W. C. Willett, "Caffeine, moderate alcohol intake, and risk of fractures of the hip and forearm in middle-aged women," *Am J Clin Nutr*, 54:1 (1991), pp. 157–63; M. A. Hansen, K. Overgaard, B. J. Riis, and C. Christiansen, "Potential risk factors for development of postmenopausal osteoporosis—examined over a 12-year period," *Osteoporosis International*, 1:2 (1991), pp. 95–102; E. A. Krall and B. Dawson-Hughes, "Smoking and bone loss among postmenopausal women," *J Bone and Mineral Research*, 6:4 (1991), pp. 331–38.

p. 214 "more frequent falls": D. D. Bikle, H. K. Genant, C. Cann, R. R. Recker, B. P. Halloran, and G. J. Strewler, "Bone disease in alcohol abuse," *Ann Intern Med*, vol. 103 (1985), pp. 42–48; M. Hernandez-Avila, et al., "Caffeine, moderate alcohol intake, and risk of fractures."

p. 214 "caffeinated drinks a day": D. P. Kiel, D. T. Felson, M. T. Hannan, J. J. Anderson, and P. W. Wilson, "Caffeine and the risk of hip fracture: the Framingham Study," *Am J Epidemiol*, 132:4 (1990), pp. 675–84.

pp. 214 "high in phosphorus": R. R. Bell, H. H. Draper, D. Y. M. Tszeng, H. K. Shin, and G. R. Schmidt, "Physiological responses of human adults to foods containing phosphate additives," *J Nutr*, vol. 107 (1977), pp. 42–50; H. H. Draper and C. A. Scythes, "Calcium, phosphorus, and osteoporosis," *Federation Proc*, 40:9 (1981), pp. 2434–38.

p. 214 "excrete more calcium": J. Reichenberg-Ullman, "Menopause naturally," *Natural Health*, Mar./Apr. 1992, p. 78.

p. 214 "negative calcium balance": R. M. Walker and H. M. Linkswiler, "Calcium retention in the adult human male as affected by protein intake," 102:10 (1972).

p. 214 "than nonvegetarians": A. G. Marsh, T. V. Sanchez, O. Mickelsen, J. Keiser, and G. Mayor, "Cortical bone density of adult lacto-ovo-vegetarian and omnivorous women," *J Am Dietetic Assn*, 76:2 (1980).

p. 214 "of bone fractures": B. J. Abelow, T. R. Holford, and K. L. Insogna, "Cross-cultural association between dietary animal protein and hip fracture: a hypothesis," *Calcified Tissue Int'l*, 50:1 (1992).

p. 214 "with a similar diet": R. Smith, "Epidemiologic studies of osteoporosis in women of Puerto Rico and Southeastern Michigan with special reference to age, race, national origin and to other related or associated findings," *Clin Orthop*, vol. 45 (1966), p. 31.

p. 214 "animal flesh is low": A. Walker, "The human requirement of calcium: Should low intakes be supplemented?" *Am J Clin Nutr*, vol. 25 (1972), p. 518; G. Lewinnek, "The significance and a comparative analysis of the epidemiology of hip fractures," *Clin Ortho Related Res*, vol. 152 (1980), p. 35; Food balance sheets, 1979–1981 average, Food and Agriculture Organization of the United Nations, Rome, 1984; FAO production yearbook, vol. 37 (1984), p. 263.

p. 215 "in the same community": J. Hu, X. Zhao, J. Jia, B. Parpia, and T. C. Campbell, "Dietary calcium and bone density among middle aged and elderly women in China," *Am J Clin Nutr* (in press).

p. 215 "of the United States": J. A. McDougall, *McDougall's Medicine: A Challenging Second Opinion* (Clinton, NJ: New Win, 1985), p. 83.

p. 215 "positive calcium balance": C. D. Arnaud and S. D. Sanchez, "The role of calcium in osteoporosis," *An Rev Nutr*, vol. 10 (1990), p. 405.

p. 216 " 'no dairy products' ": J. Hu, X. Zhao, J. Chen, B. Parpia, and T. C. Campbell, "Associations between daily nutrient intake, flesh food consumption and bone mass of pre- and post-menopausal women," *FASEB J*, 6:5 (1992), paper no. 4951.

p. 217 "tends to be more expensive": "Choosing a calcium supplement," *Health After 50* (Feb. 1991), p. 3.

p. 218 "your last period": B. Ettinger: "Benefits of long term hormone replacement therapy," personal communication. Unpublished paper.

Chapter 11

p. 222 "porcupine and monkey": H. A. Junod, *The Life of a South African Tribe*, vol. 2 (London: Macmillan, 1927), p. 185.

p. 222 "powers of their husbands": L. J. Pospisil, *Kapauku Papuans and Their Law* (New Haven: Yale University Press, 1958), p. 59; M. J. Levy, *The Family Revolution in Modern China* (Cambridge, MA: Harvard University Press, 1949), p. 129.

p. 222 "men have been given": J. Griffen, "A cross-cultural investigation of behavioral changes at menopause," *Soc Sci J*, 14:2 (1977), p. 52.

p. 222 "until after menopause": Ibid., p. 51.

p. 223　"and healing powers": Ibid., p. 53.

p. 223　"meaningfully *on her*": M. M. Buck and L. N. Gottlieb, "The meaning of time: Mohawk women at midlife," *Health Care for Women Int'l*, 12:1 (1991), p. 41.

p. 226　"increase in some women": L. Speroff, R. Glass, and N. Kase, *Clinical Gynecologic Endocrinology and Infertility* (Baltimore, MD: Williams and Wilkins, 1989), p. 128.

p. 226　"In one study": "Empty Nest Syndrome," *Regarding Women and Healthcare*, Fall 1989, p. 1.

p. 227　"stage of life": L. Banner, "The meaning of menopause: Aging and historical contexts in the twentieth century," Working paper #3, University of Wisconsin, Center for 20th Century Studies, 1989/90, p. 25.

p. 228　*"Most Valuable Asset"*: S. Johnson, *One Minute for Myself: How to Manage Your Most Valuable Asset* (New York: Avon, 1987).

p. 231　"symptoms during menopause: A. A. Haspels and H. Musaph, "Psychosexual aspects of mid-life," in P. A. Van Keep, W. H. Utian, and A. Vermeulen (eds.), *The Controversial Climacteric* (Lancaster, England: MTP Press, 1982).

p. 231　"at menopause clinics": M. I. Whitehead, "The menopause. Part A: hormone 'replacement' therapy—the controversies," in L. Dennerstein and G. Burrows (eds.), *Handbook of Psychosomatic Obstetrics and Gynaecology* (New York: Elsevier, 1983).

Epilogue

p. 236　"seek medical treatment": G. Cowdan, L. Warren, and J. Young, "Medical perceptions of menopausal symptoms," *Psychol Women Quart*, vol. 9 (1985), pp. 3–14.

p. 237　"their symptoms debilitating": B. M. Barbo, "The physiology of the menopause," *Medical Clinics of North America*, 71:1 (1987), p. 11.

p. 240　"read *Mainstay*": M. Strong, *Mainstay: For the Well Spouse of the Chronically Ill* (New York: Penguin, 1988).

p. 243　"to mid-fifties": D. J. Levinson, *The Seasons of a Man's Life* (New York: Ballantine, 1978).

p. 248　"became most important": *Longevity*, Feb. 1992.